A UNIQUE BOOK

Parents will here find practical advice about their child's bowel disorders—what to do about them, when to call the doctor.

There is hard-to-find information that can save travelers and campers from the acute discomfort of stomach upsets and diarrhea.

Adults and the elderly will benefit from Dr. Troy's counsel about diet, exercise and cleanliness. The simple treatments suggested for constipation have relieved even chronic sufferers after drugs have failed. Find out exactly what brand-name products can be safely used—or *not* used—and for which problems.

For the continuing health of you and your family, keep Dr. Troy's book as a handy reference. You'll be rewarded with greater comfort—and a healthier digestion!

BETTER BOWEL HEALTH

Dr. Marian T. Troy

M.B., B.S., FR.C.S.(C)., F.A.C.S.

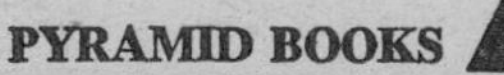
PYRAMID BOOKS NEW YORK

BETTER BOWEL HEALTH

A PYRAMID BOOK

First printing, December 1974

ISBN 0-515-03572-6

Library of Congress Catalog Card Number: 74-24436

Printed in the United States of America

Pyramid Books are published by Pyramid Communications, Inc. Its trademarks, consisting of the word "Pyramid" and the portrayal of a pyramid, are registered in the United States Patent Office.

PYRAMID COMMUNICATIONS, INC.
919 Third Avenue
New York, New York 10022, U.S.A.

This is to thank my wife, Margaret, for her help with the editing of this book, for supplying ideas for a section on food recipes, and, above all, for putting up with me while I wrote it.

Dr. Marian Troy

Calgary, Alberta

Contents

1. The Story of Waterloo

On the morning of June 18, 1815, near the small Belgian town of Waterloo, Napoleon Bonaparte faced two problems. One was the combined British, Belgian, Prussian, and Netherlands army of the Duke of Wellington. His other problem was hemorrhoids.

Napoleon's opponent, the Duke of Wellington, spent the morning nervously pacing up and down, scanning his maps, dispatching one messenger after another. A crack Prussian contingent commanded by Field Marshal Gebhard von Blücher was missing, delayed somewhere in the Belgian countryside. The Allies' chances were slim.

Napoleon knew that his army should attack early that day, before the Iron Duke's forces had had a chance to dig in, and certainly before the Prussians could arrive on the scene. But he could not do it. He had diarrhea. His hemorrhoids were prolapsed. He could not even sit on a horse, much less command an army. So he tended to his sore posterior. The chances of a French victory rushed away with every change of water from his sitz bath. By midafternoon his personal surgeons succeeded in patching him up, a bit. He gave the order to charge. But it was too late. The battle raged until evening, its outcome in the balance. Then, Blücher's forces arrived and tipped the scale. Victory went to the Allies.

After his defeat at Waterloo, Napoleon never again

was able to raise another army. French forces in distant North America became demoralized. A large proportion of them were withdrawn back to France. The remainder engaged in, and lost, a series of battles against the British. French influence waned. The British claimed all of the New World as a colony. The English language came to stay. English customs prevailed.

Today you do not usually drink wine with your food. Your daily meals are not classed as cuisine. Except in Louisiana and Quebec, the laws that govern your work and play are based on the old English Common Law of Precedents, not on the Roman and Canon laws of the Code Civil. That marvelous French plumbing invention, the bidet—designed, as it was, especially for the efficient cleansing of a saddle-sore posterior, as well as for the treatment of so many anorectal disorders—never caught on here. Pity.

A healthy digestion is well-being, is ability to work and play, is contentment, is money in the bank, is happiness. Without it your outlook on life is soured, your work performance suffers, you lose sleep and money, you fight with your spouse, or you take it out on your children. You cannot concentrate. You cannot even talk about it. It isn't polite. You suffer in silence and try this remedy or that; you fall for one advertisement after another. You worry about diet; you imagine possible complications. While you are worrying, your gastrointestinal function keeps getting worse. And worse.

The purpose of this book is, first, to tell you what a normal digestion is all about—how to attain it if it is attainable for you, how to prevent disturbances if possible, how to manage and remedy some of them if they do occur, how to recognize serious symptoms early. A normal intestinal function is attainable for just about everybody. The rules are simple. Following them is enjoyable. Success is easy.

One word of caution. This book is not a do-it-yourself medical guide; it is not designed to take the place of a doctor. It is rather intended to supplement, and to explain, what a doctor would normally advise. Of necessity, and for the sake of completeness, this book mentions drugs. All drugs have disadvantages. Some are dangerous. As far as possible, the drawbacks of all drug treatments are mentioned whenever applicable. Never take *any* drugs without consulting your doctor, first.

Part I. The Intestinal Tract

2. Introduction

The intestinal tract starts at the lips and ends at the anus. In between it consists of a long fleshy tube that looks simple but serves fantastically complicated and wonderfully integrated structures and functions.

The lips serve as the gate to the digestive system. The texture of potential food items is checked here for obvious evidence of edibility or nonedibility. In addition, the lips have some taste function and on the inside bear small salivary glands that secrete saliva, or spit. The function of the teeth is obvious: The front teeth, called incisors, serve to bite off or tear off mouth-size chunks of food; the side teeth, or molars, grind the food into smaller particles, which are then swallowed. Saliva from many small salivary glands on the inside of the cheeks, as well as from six large salivary glands, moistens the food and starts digestion by breaking down some of the constituents of food—notably starches—into chemically somewhat different compounds. Farther along in the intestinal tract, these compounds will be further acted upon by other digestive juices until every food substance is changed into chemical compounds able to pass through the walls of the intestine into the blood, then carried to the liver, and eventually carried to every tissue in the body.

The tongue has very important functions besides gossiping. It pushes food around the mouth into the grinding mill that is made up of the molars; it mixes the food with saliva and with the water or other liquid you take with your meals. It feels the ground-up food and determines when it is chewed enough for swallowing without choking. Finally, it propels the food backward to the flap valve called the glottis.

The glottis separates the trachea (windpipe) from the pharynx (back of the mouth). The back of the tongue and the glottis act in conjunction most of the time. If their coordination is ever defective, such as may happen when you try to talk at the same time as you try to swallow, then the food may go "down the wrong way." This may have happened to you at some time. It is not pleasant.

Food next passes through the esophagus (foodpipe), which leads from the back of the throat through the chest and diaphragm into the stomach. It is not just a passive ride. The act of swallowing is a complex function in which waves of muscular contraction of the esophagus actively propel food and drink along the way. It is possible—for some people at least—to eat and even to drink while standing on their head. The waves of contractions that make such defiance of gravity possible are called peristalsis.

The stomach proper is a widened area of the long intestinal tube and is situated in the upper part of the abdomen, in the midline and just to the left of the midline, right under the diaphragm and the ribcage. Many people incorrectly call stomach everything that lies between the ribs above and the pelvis below. The proper name for the part of the body that contains the stomach, liver, spleen, pancreas, and all of the intestines is abdomen. You might also call it the belly. If large, it deserves the name paunch.

The stomach proper serves as a reservoir, or storage area. Here a whole meal is initially accommodated. It is quite capacious; hors d'oeuvres, soup, meat, potatoes, vegetables, gravy and dumplings, dessert, coffee and liquor—all are stored here. Obviously, however, there are limits as to how much it can hold. If you overeat, your stomach tells you about it and will con-

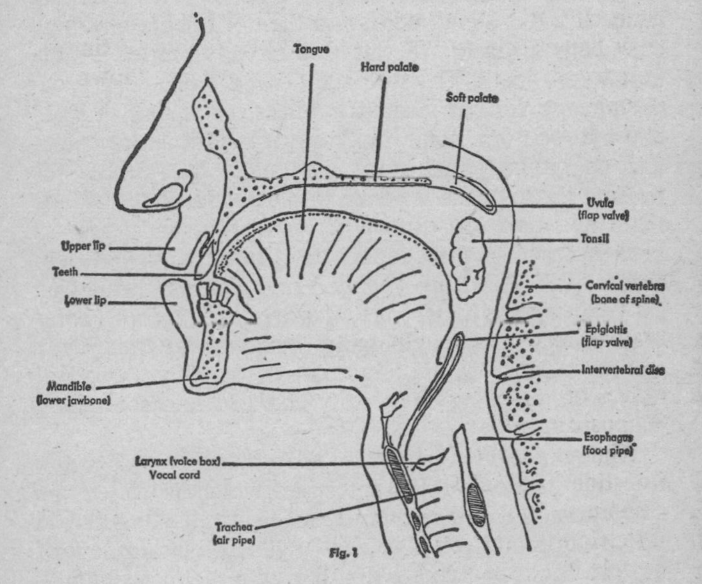

Fig. 1. During swallowing two flap valves prevent food going "the wrong way." The soft palate and uvula shut off the posterior passage to the nose cavity. The epiglottis shuts off the passage through the larynx (voice box) to the trachea (air pipe).

tinue to tell you about it until a substantial part of the meal has moved along to the next part of the intestinal tube, called the duodenum. When your stomach is empty, it also tells you about that sad state of affairs; it growls and contracts and churns. The sensation you experience is hunger.

Digestion of food consists first of the breaking up of pieces and chunks into smaller pieces, next of mixing them with digestive juices, and then of further churning them into a mash. All this was already started by the mouth and teeth. The stomach takes the churning process a stage further. Stomach juices, principally pepsin and hydrochloric acid, break down the food into chemical compounds that must eventually be suitable for passing through the walls of the intestine. Protein—the main nutritive constituent of meat, fish, and eggs—is broken down in the stomach to substances called peptones. Milk solids are changed into caseins. Swallowed saliva continues to act here. It works on starches (potatoes, bakery goods), changing them into dextrins. Only alcohol—beer, wines, liquors—is actually absorbed here without being chemically changed into something else.

Once the food mash leaves the stomach it passes into the first portion of the intestine, which is called the duodenum. The name literally means twelve fingers laid side by side and refers to the length of that segment of the gut. Most people are familiar with the duodenum—some unfortunately more so than they care, because the duodenum is subject to the disease of peptic duodenal ulceration. Additional digestive juices enter here through two separate ducts: one from the pancreas (sweetbread), which carries pancreatic juice; the other from the liver, which carries bile.

Pancreatic juice acts further on the proteins, which had already been partly broken down in the stomach into proteoses and peptones, changing them chemically into polypeptides and various amino acids. Pancreatic juice also acts on ingested fats, turning them into glycerol and fatty acids, and continues the action of saliva

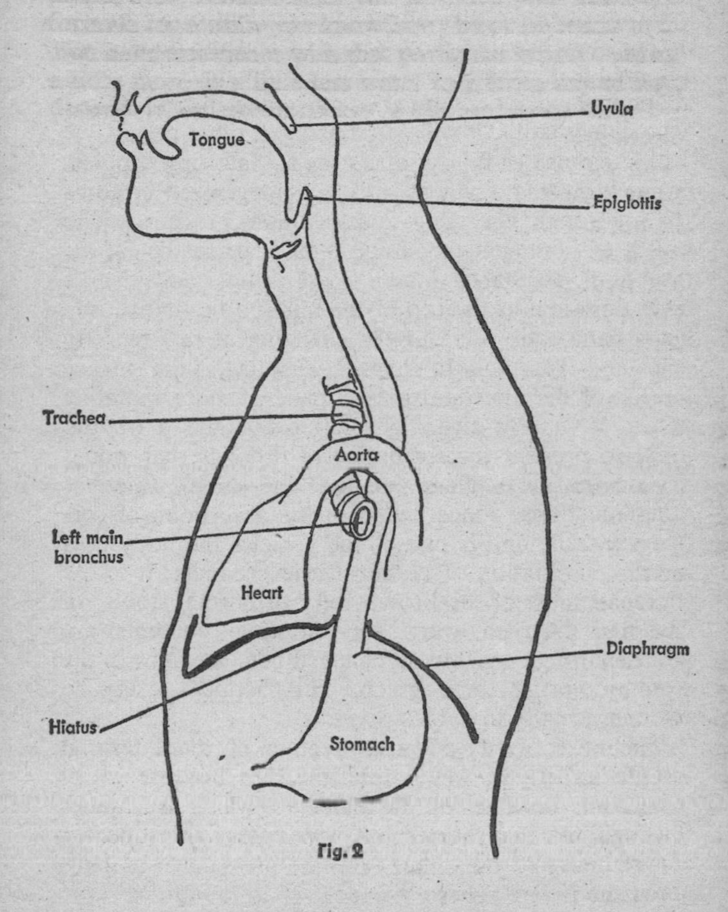

Fig. 2. The esophagus (food pipe) passes through the chest cavity and through a muscular dome which is the diaphragm, and enters the stomach. The spot where it pierces the diaphragm is called the esophageal hiatus.

on starches, turning them into maltose, among other things.

All in all, apart from stomach juice pancreatic juice is the most powerful and most important of all digestive juices. Only the pancreas itself and the duodenum can hold it. If it spills out of these "containers" into the abdominal cavity in the process of the disease called acute pancreatitis, it will actually digest other organs.

Bile emulsifies fats: it disperses fat into tiny droplets in much the same way as milk is homogenized by forcing it through very tiny nozzles under pressure. (The object of homogenizing milk is to disperse the fat all through it, so that it does not rise up and collect as a layer of cream at the top of the milk bottle.) Next, bile helps pancreatic juice in the changing of fats to fatty acids and eventually to soaps. It also lowers the surface tension of the intestinal mash (makes it more wettable, just as a window-cleaning solution contains a wetting agent to prevent the formation of droplets that would dry on the clean glass and mar the shine). Bile has other functions, concerned with the absorption of certain vitamins, and is one of the vehicles the body uses for the elimination of certain waste products. It is the source of most of the brown color of normal stools. In cases of diarrhea when the intestinal contents are rushed through quickly, unchanged bile can show in the stools, coloring them green. This happens every so often, especially in babies.

The next twenty-odd-foot section of the intestinal tract is called the small intestine, not because of its length but because of its diameter, which is smaller than that of the shorter but wider large intestine (or colon). Parts of the small intestine are known as jejunum and ileum. These are not separate entities. One merges into the other.

The function of the small intestine is the absorption of food nutrients, which is accomplished through a rather complicated mechanism. The inside lining of the intestine is studded with a very large number of tiny structures called villi, each of which is richly supplied with blood vessels. Each villus is bathed in the nutrient mash, which passes through the lumen of the bowel. What was steak and baked potato and green beans and apple pie at the mouth level is now, thanks to all the digestive juices that have acted upon it, a complex mixture of organic chemicals. The digestive system to this point is thus a chemical factory, the end products of which now soak through, or diffuse, into the cells lining the villi, where they are picked up by the blood. The blood transports all these nourishment chemicals first to the liver for storage; then, as the need arises, all over the body.

There are a few bacteria in the small intestine. They act on carbohydrates (starches), causing fermentation and thus contributing a small amount of intestinal gas. Most of the gas in the intestine consists of swallowed air.

The small intestine terminates in the large intestine, otherwise known as the colon, at a point near the right groin. The appendix is attached exactly where the two join. By the time the intestinal mash has reached here, about all of its nutrient substances have been extracted. What remain and pass into the colon are water and food residues: cellulose from vegetable matter; keratin from the connective tissues of meat; magnesium, calcium, and other poorly absorbed salts; some iron; residues of bile; hard pieces of bone or gristle swallowed with meat; and hopefully most of the artificial coloring matter and other food additives that food processors have added to their products. In addition, there comes through here the air swallowed while eating or drinking, some fermentation by-products such as hydrogen gas and hydrogen sulfide gas, some cholesterol shed off intestinal lining cells, and mucus.

In the colon there happily live a large number of bacteria, most of which do you no harm whatever but help move colon contents along by digesting and fermenting, in part by putrefying some of the food residues that the small intestine has disdained. These bacteria, by the way, do you no harm *only* as long as they stay where

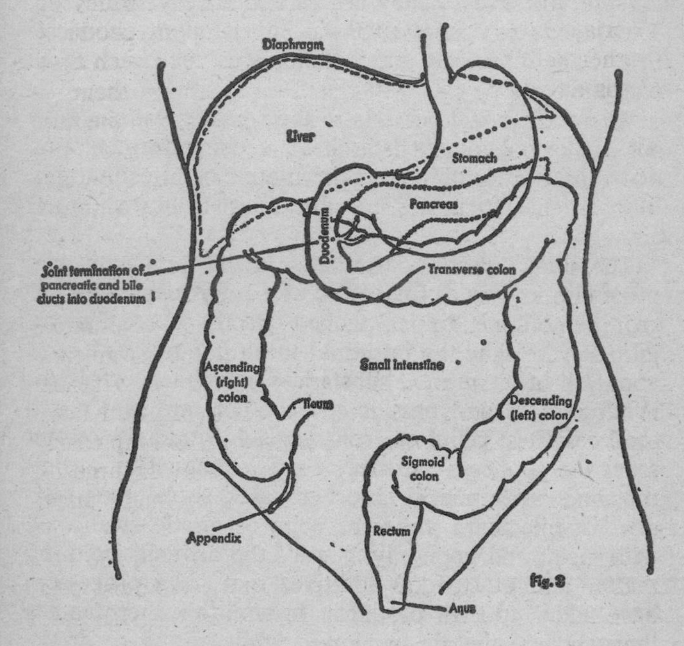

Fig. 3. The intestinal tract.

they belong—in the colon. If you should get these bacteria into your mouth—either by not washing your hands after using the toilet and then chewing your fingernails, or by drinking water contaminated with sewage—then they could do you much harm indeed.

The functions of the colon are, first, absorption of water and some minerals; second, excretion of some poisons and waste products from the blood; third, fermentation and putrefaction of some food residues by bacteria; and fourth, storage of all these waste products together with bacteria and intestinal gas until such time as it is necessary and convenient to eliminate them.

The leftovers of your Sunday dinner arrive in the first part of the colon, called the cecum, about four or five hours after you have finished the coffee and desert. They move along to the hepatic flexure, the first bend of the colon situated on the upper right side of your abdomen, some six or seven hours after eating. They take a further three hours or so to traverse the part of the colon across the upper abdomen to the bend situated in the left upper corner of your tummy called the splenic flexure, then take an additional three hours to reach the sigmoid, or pelvic part of the colon situated near your left groin. There they lie immobilized for up to six or even eight hours. By the time you have an urge to evacuate, some eighteen to twenty-two hours have elapsed from the time the food was eaten.

Thus, with a normal, undisturbed digestion, the appearance of stools reflect what was eaten almost one whole day earlier. In cases of diarrhea the passage time is much accelerated; in constipation it is delayed.

The absorption of water from the colon is a slow business. If the passage of stools is rapid, then much water fails to become absorbed. Thus, diarrhea stools are watery. In constipation the stool stays in the colon longer, there is more time for more thorough absorption of water, and the longer the interval between evacuations, the drier and harder and more compacted will the stool be. It follows that in the treatment of diarrhea the water lost in the stools must be replaced either by drinking or, if this is not possible, by giving the water intravenously. In the treatment of constipation extra water must be taken with all meals and also between meals—not for the sake of the needs of the whole body but in order to keep the stools soft and the evacuation reasonably easy.

3. What Is Normal

Persephone, the ancient Greek goddess of flowers, once walked in a lush green meadow and, singing gaily, gathered flowers for a wreath. Along came Pluto, the god of the underworld, in his black chariot. He fell in love with the beautiful Persephone. Courtship customs being rough in those days, he did not pause to ask her wishes but simply kidnapped her and carried her away to his nether kingdom. There he planned to make her his queen.

Persephone, however, did not like this at all. Among the treasures of natural gas, and oil, and all the other resources over which Pluto was boss, she missed her wholesome, balanced diet of grains, nuts, fruit, and milk. Pluto could not supply such a diet to her. The larder of his black palace of coal and aluminum and copper and iron was paneled with gold and studded with precious stones. There were riches all around that would make any president of any natural resource company green with envy. But all there was for Persephone to eat were pomegranate seeds. Poor Persephone's digestion suffered terribly.

In the meantime, on the surface of the earth, there was no one to tend to established flowers or to plant new ones. All existing plantlife gradually died. The weather grew cold. Winter set in.

Finally Pluto could not stand to see the suffering of his bride any longer. He allowed her to return to the surface of the earth for six-month periods of time, during which she not only attended to her digestion but also walked joyously across the fields and meadows, while crocuses and snowdrops and daisies and buttercups sprang up all around her feet. Thus ended the first winter and came the first spring.

The Oxford Dictionary defines "normal" as conforming to a standard, or usual, or regular. The "ideal" digestion would be one that never, never gives any trouble whatever. Even a Greek goddess did not have it. Chances are that you do not have it either. Chances are that from time to time you, like everybody else, at times experience problems, usually produced by eating something that does not agree with you. Chances are that once you, like Persephone, get back to eating a balanced diet, your digestive troubles improve.

The symptoms of digestive disturbances are known to everyone. They include nausea, bad breath, heartburn, vomiting, various abnormal abdominal sensations, pain, diarrhea, constipation, flatulence. This book attempts to deal with the causes of the most common symptoms. Your doctor investigates your ailments by listening to your story, by examining you, and additionally by having you undergo various tests and x-rays. Nine-tenths of digestive illnesses can be diagnosed first by knowing what is the normal or average and second by recognizing what is not. Important clues are furnished by observing the function of the lower bowel (intestine) at various ages.

The intestinal tract of the newborn baby contains a dark brown, almost black, ointmentlike substance called meconium. This is derived partly from bile and partly from mucous secretions of the developing intestine. Mixed with it are surface cells shed by the intestinal lining. The normal infant usually passes his or her first meconium stool within ten hours after birth. The first few stools are black. As the baby is fed, meconium stools become transitional in appearance. They become first greenish brown and may contain undigested milk curds. Later they become greenish yellow from digested milk; finally, by the end of the first week of life they assume the typical golden yellow appearance and salve-like consistency of babyhood. They may still contain seedlike particles of congealed milk curds, called bird-seed stools. They either have no smell or smell faintly acid. They are never offensive.

The stools of a breast-fed baby are always a little looser in consistency than those of an infant fed cows' milk. The frequency of bowel movements varies tremendously: the average breast-fed infant has two to four stools a day. The average formula-fed infant has one or two stools per day. It happens that an infant may have only one stool in two or three or, exceptionally, every four days. If the infrequent stool is soft and pasty and salve-like and golden-yellow, and if the baby is otherwise healthy—is not vomiting and his or her tummy is not swelling—then this tardiness is not abnormal. No treatment is necessary.

Undigested milk curds in the stools are recognized as yellow- or brownish-coated nodules that, when broken, contain a white, caseinlike substance. Generally they are of no significance; if too numerous, they may be a cause of constipation. The milk curds of breast-fed babies are always smaller, less numerous, and softer and never cause constipation.

Tiny white lumps in diarrheal stools of babies are not milk curds but undigested fat.

As the baby starts to crawl, turns into a toddler, and eats more varied food, his or her stools become firmer and darker and acquire an odor. By the end of the first year of life one stool per day is the rule. Again, there are exceptions. If the stools are soft and formed and are not hard or lumpy or dry, and if the child does not exhibit any signs of ill health, a bowel movement every second or third day is nothing to be alarmed about.

The stools of children from the age of two years on

resemble adult stools in all respects. Mothers are frequently amazed at the size of the stools these youngsters produce. All this means only that young tissues are wonderfully elastic and eminently stretchable. Unless there are other symptoms, this is definitely no cause for worry.

Older children, teenagers, and adults usually have one bowel movement daily, but many people habitually have two. In the latter case, the combined volumes of the two daily movements amount to more than is passed by people who have one evacuation per day. The twice-daily stool is also softer because it takes time for the colon to extract water from food residue, and the quicker the passage time, the less water is absorbed and the bulkier and more watery is the stool. With a once-daily evacuation, the total daily amount passed roughly corresponds to the capacity of the individual's descending colon, that is, to the capacity of the bowel from the left (or splenic) flexure, located just under the left rib margin, to the rectum. A large man who is a heavy eater will produce more stools daily than a child or a small woman. The total weight of daily stools varies with the size of the individual, the amounts of indigestible roughage eaten, and the amount of water contained in them.

The normal adult stool is soft, yet formed, with the consistency of a thick paste. The normal color is various shades of brown, anything from honey maple to dark oak or mahogany, depending upon the diet the previous day. High protein—that is, mostly meat—diets produce a dark stool. Diets rich in milk and other dairy foods give light-colored stools. The normal odor is unpleasant but not foul.

In older age, when all body functions slow down, the intestinal tract likewise tends to act sluggishly. Because the stool stays longer in the colon, more water is extracted and the evacuation of the average older person tends to be harder and drier; the volume is less. This by itself does not necessarily constitute constipation. As is the case in children and adults, a pattern of reasonably regular evacuations every three to four days is, by itself, nothing to worry about. Constipation, by definition, is a condition in which the stools are not only hard and dry but also difficult to pass. Constipation does, however, occur fairly often in old age. This subject is discussed more fully in Section 51.

4. What Is Not Normal

Noticing gross changes from normal digestion patterns is easy. Severe pain, persistent nausea, and debilitating diarrhea are symptoms that alarm anyone. For timely spotting of developing disease, it pays to know what to look for, early.

Look at your stools before flushing them down. Like the exhaust fumes of a car, their appearance tells you a great deal about your digestive mechanism. The easiest abnormality to spot in stools is blood. If you do notice blood in the toilet bowl, then also make a mental note of whether the blood is bright cherry red or dull red-brown or almost black. Blood changes color while being transported in the digestive tract. The longer it is in the bowel, the darker it becomes. Bright red blood always originates from the anus or rectum. The darker it is, the farther up is the bleeding point.

Estimate how much blood there is: just a smear on the toilet paper, a teaspoon, a cupful, a quart, or even more. Notice, if you can, if the blood comes with the stool or mainly with the straining before the stool, or mostly afterward; whether it comes in driplets or in a solid stream. The commonest cause of driplet bleeding with and following the stool is hemorrhoids. Blood mixed with the stool usually originates from a polyp but can also originate from diverticulosis or a cancer. Massive dark red or black bleeding most commonly comes from an ulcer of the stomach or duodenum. The stool in these cases also has a very offensive smell. It is called a melena stool.

Every case of rectal bleeding should be investigated by a doctor. The more you are able to tell your doctor about the characteristics of the bleeding, the quicker he will be able to reach a diagnosis and institute the necessary treatment.

Notice the color of the stool itself. Is it a normal brown shading from light tan to deep mahogany or oak, or is the color really strange—such as green or yellow or jet black? Green stools occur with diarrhea, especially in babies (see Section 9). Yellow or orange stools indicate that insufficient bile is mixed with the intestinal contents, as happens in some types of liver disease or biliary disease and may be the first sign of jaundice. Slate gray and blackish stools are frequently caused by iron medication taken in the treatment of anemia. Iron is also one of the constituents of many tonics. Very dark olive blue or olive gray "smeary" stools with a grossly offensive odor indicate excessive putrefaction, usually the result of a meal or a diet too rich in both protein and fat. Jet black, offensive melena stools, mentioned already, indicate severe bleeding high in the intestinal tract, usually from an ulcer in the stomach or duodenum, but can also occur from swallowing blood from a massive nosebleed, or following a tooth extraction.

Notice how much stool is there—the normal amount as described already or much more or considerably less. Do the stools sink in the toilet bowl, or do they float? Do they look greasy? Overfat stools that float on water are a sign of certain diseases of the pancreas and of certain disorders of metabolism. They signify that the fat eaten in the diet has not been digested.

Is the consistency of the stools habitually mushy or frothy? If so, excessive fermentation is taking place. Diet starches are not being absorbed properly. The diet is probably too rich in carbohydrates. Conversely, are the stools unusually hard and dry and difficult to pass? This is true constipation.

All these observations are easy to make. All are important and can help you to get a good idea of the nature of your digestive troubles. If necessary, your doctor will be able to interpret your findings further.

5. Changes in Digestive Habits Can Mean Cancer

Digestive habits are conditioned by a multiplicity of factors such as heredity, childhood experiences, psychologic experiences, diet, exercise, general health, presence of constitutional or chronic disorders, past illnesses, cultural influences. Once they are reasonably established, unless there is a drastic change in health or mode of living, they become the habits of a lifetime. A child who has never had any significant problems with stomach upsets, heartburn, bloating, cramps, or bowel disturbances is not likely to develop these symptoms as an adult, unless there is a reason.

I am not now speaking of transitory changes. If Johnny gets into the neighbor's garden and fills his stomach with stolen apples, then he will deserve, and will surely get, a bout of diarrhea. If you yourself take an airline trip to Mexico or Japan and first spend hours sitting cramped in an airplane seat stuffing your face and your stomach, then on arrival proceed to celebrate the occasion with more unaccustomed food spiked with tequila or sake, you will likewise deserve, and will get, first a bout of acute flatulence, then constipation, then diarrhea. But if, on the other hand, you do neither of these exciting things but spend your life working to pacify the mortgage company and the Internal Revenue Service and if you have always had a stomach that seemed to be lined with stainless steel and a set of intestines that were able to deal with almost any abuse yet find yourself either rapidly *or gradually* shopping for indigestion relievers or laxatives or antidiarrhea remedies, then watch out.

This book does not deal with all illnesses that influence digestion patterns. It does not deal with disorders of other organs, such as glands, blood and blood-forming organs, chest, brain, or heart. Disorders of the liver, of the biliary tract, and of the pancreas are mentioned only briefly. A change from established digestive habits can be caused by numerous disorders of any number of body systems. Or it can be caused by cancer.

Cancer is not a single disease but a large group of diseases. All cancers have in common a disorganization of the body's ability to repair itself and to grow. In cancer, cells—which previously were quietly and contentedly serving their humble function, each a minuscule part of some organ—suddenly desert their duties and abandon themselves to an unbridled population explosion. Usually, in the early stages of cancer development, this rapid reproduction results in the cells growing tightly together, heaped upon one another. Thus, the first sign of cancer is the development of a nodule or mass or lump. The lump behaves as a parasite. It lives on, but does not contribute to, the work of the tissue it afflicts. Thus, the first effect of an early cancer is interference with the function of the organ from which it has arisen.

Because the tissue that makes up a cancer is growing

in a disorganized fashion, it frequently does not have a covering of surface cells. Blood vessels mixed haphazardly within it also grow on the surface of it, where they are subject to abrasion. Consequently another early sign of cancer is bleeding. The abraded surface is liable to become infected. The result is ulceration, which furnishes the fourth early sign of cancer: a mucoid and purulent and bloody discharge.

It is a truism that for cancer treatment to be successful it must begin early. Like all truisms, it too does not hold in every case. Some few cancers will progress in spite of early treatment; conversely, there are many instances where late treatment is effective. But generally the statement is valid.

Cancers of the lips, tongue, and pharynx (the food passage part of the throat) first show themselves by the appearance of a nonpainful, nontender small lump. Cancers of the esophagus (foodpipe) show their early presence by a vague, ill-defined sensation of something interfering with swallowing. Food seems to take longer to go down or to pause or to stick. At times, only the swallowing of some types of food or drink gives this sensation.

Cancers of the stomach give diverse early signs, none of which is prominent, few of which usually include pain. There may be a feeling of fullness or of satiety, so that the person is just not hungry and often loses weight. There may be a change in appetite—some previously favorite foods may now seem tasteless or taste differently. There may be slight nausea, a kind of prolonged morning-after feeling, a vague, indistinct sensation of there being something different. Similar symptoms also occur in cases of plain old stomach upsets (gastritis), gastroenteritis, peptic ulceration, gall bladder disease, and in hepatitis. The important thing to notice about them is whether they have occurred previously, whether they develop along the lines typical of these other diseases, and whether they persist—in other words, whether or not they amount to a change in accustomed digestive patterns. Accompanying them there may also develop a change in accustomed evacuation patterns.

Primary cancers of the duodenum are so rare that for practical purposes they can be ignored. However, primary cancers of the neighboring pancreas do affect the duodenum in several ways. They may compress it, causing feelings of fullness, of an unwillingness to eat, of nausea or vomiting. Also, there may be a feeling of a nagging discomfort, not quite amounting to pain, which is felt in the upper abdomen and sometimes in the back. A pancreatic cancer may compress the bile ducts, so that liver bile does not flow freely into the duodenium. The digestion of fats is interfered with. Stools become greasy and light in color and tend to float on the surface. These signs can precede the development of jaundice.

Primary small bowel cancers are almost unheard of, but primary large bowel cancers do occur—the farther along in the large bowel, the more frequently. Large bowel (colon) cancers often are first detectable by a change in accustomed elimination patterns. The affected person experiences, for no clearly apparent reason, a loosening of the stools. This can be either constant and steady (daily) or intermittent (occurring as a series of bouts). With it, there may be feelings of urgency to move the bowels, of being unable to wait for an opportune time, of having to pass more flatus than has been customary, as well as sensations of not having emptied the bowels properly, even after apparently adequate motions. Bouts of constipation may alternate with bouts of diarrhea, especially if the affected individual resorts to self-medication with laxatives and antidiarrhea remedies.

A change—any change—in accustomed elimination patterns is suspicious. Should you experience it, do not attempt to treat it yourself. Have it checked out by your doctor.

Rectal cancers at times give rise to a sensation of fullness in the rectum, a feeling that the bowel is still full, even immediately after seemingly adequate evacuations. This feeling is apt to persist between bowel movements. A person so affected visits the bathroom more often and spends more time there than has been his or her custom previously. This sensation, called tenesmus, is a very significant early symptom, as is the discharge of mucus or blood either with or apart from bowel movements.

In concluding this section I would like to emphasize that disturbances of digestive function are very, very common, while cancers of the digestive tract are not. If you experience any of the symptoms described above, do not immediately jump to the conclusion that you have cancer. Read elsewhere in this book to see if your symptoms more closely fit something else. Decide if there is, perhaps, a clear reason for your problems; a change in diet can have done it, or a change in the mode of living, or nervous tension, or worry. If you cannot think of a clear reason for the change, then play it safe. See your doctor soon.

Part II. Diarrhea

6. Introduction

Diarrhea is the abnormally rapid evacuation of intestinal contents. It is a symptom of disease; it is not a disease in itself. This point is important both in diagnosis and in treatment. In serious cases the cause must always be recognized first, before intelligent treatment can be given. If you compare diarrhea to a flood of water cascading through your home, the source and cause of the stream must first be identified, then the broken pipe mended or the hole in the roof stopped up, before the damage to ceilings and rugs can be assessed and repaired.

Treating the symptom alone has its place when the cause cannot be readily recognized. Doing so is like throwing sawdust on the stream of water cascading down your bedroom stairs or placing pans on the floor to collect the drips from the ceiling. It prevents further damage to the house while giving you time to locate the burst pipe between the wall joists.

The human body has its own built-in repair capability. Most of the time you do not have to wait for the plumber. Consequently symptomatic treatment has a very important place in medicine. Most cases of diarrhea can be treated symptomatically, as can many other passing ailments such as colds, coughs, headaches, some fevers, and most "rheumatic" aches and pains. The body will look after the treatment of the underlying condition itself.

At least 90 percent of cases of diarrhea fall into this category. The underlying illness is short-lived, transient, self-limiting. Even in that vast majority of instances it helps to have an idea of what has caused the trouble and to correct or remove such cause if feasible. In the remaining less than 10 percent of cases the illness causing the diarrhea is serious. The body may not be able to deal with it unaided. The diarrhea may persist and may damage the organism seriously. Very acute diarrhea or long-persistent diarrhea is a grave and life-threatening condition. If this should happen to you, or especially if it should happen to your child, then get in touch with your doctor with no further delay.

7. Diarrhea—What Actually Happens

The mechanism of propulsion of the food mash through the twenty-odd feet of the intestine is called peristalsis. It is described in more detail in Section 32. It is produced by alternate contractions and relaxations of layers of muscles within the walls of the intestine, which serve to squeeze segments of the bowel, and to milk the contents along. There is normally a phase of relaxation of a bowel segment, followed by a wave of contraction, the two following each other in slow, orderly sequence. In diarrhea there is always some agent or cause that irritates the bowel. The peristaltic rushes become fast, violent, and disorganized. Contraction waves work against each other and may cause the backing up of intestinal contents, so that vomiting occurs. The violence of the contractions accounts for the cramps, spasms, rushes, gurgles, and squeaks with which any sufferer is so familiar.

The typical diarrhea stool is thin and watery and frequent. It breaks apart in the water of the toilet bowl. If diarrhea is severe, then the stool looks in all respects just like colored water with few coherent particles. Such stool is definitely abnormal and indicates that your intestinal contents are rushing through you at a great speed. Very little of the food eaten is absorbed. You are actually losing more water than you have drunk. There are cramps and pain, and since the discomfort makes you swallow extra air, there is usually much gas.

The recurrent painful spasms of diarrhea are generalized: they are felt in all areas of the abdomen, although usually more so on the left side, the side of the descending or terminal portion of the colon. If the diarrhea lasts, after a while a feeling of constant (not only spasmodic) discomfort appears in addition to the cramps that still flit from side to side, up and down and across the abdomen. This constant achiness, or frank pain, is also generalized, is felt all over the abdomen. It means that the whole bowel is now inflamed—this in addition to its still experiencing the spasms and cramps of the overactive peristalsis. Yet if you now push on various parts of your abdomen with your fingers, this pressure is not by itself painful and may even be soothing.

Watch out if in pushing on various parts of your abdomen in this way, you should discover one area where the finger pressure does produce pain. The sensation of pain on pressure is called tenderness. If localized to one spot it means that there is an extra severe inflammation in that particular area. In diarrhea you can expect such tenderness on the left side, the descending colon side of the abdomen. Tenderness anywhere else spells additional trouble. Tenderness on the right lower side, anywhere above the groin and below the level of the navel, may mean appendicitis.

Other symptoms associated with diarrhea mean other things. Vomiting means either that the disease process producing the diarrhea is so severe and peristalsis so disorganized that bowel content is backing up or that the stomach as well as the intestines is involved in the disease process. This condition, called gastroenteritis, is common, especially in children. If serious, it quickly leads to a debilitating loss of body fluids and body salts called electrolytes. (More about this later, in Section 8.) The smaller the child or baby, the quicker it can develop into life-endangering illness.

Headache, an overall feeling of lassitude and debility, weakness of the whole body, irritability—all these are symptoms both of the disease producing the diarrhea and of the loss of body fluids produced by the diarrhea. The rectum and anal region become irritated and inflamed by the passage of liquid stools. Small quiescent hemorrhoids are liable to become inflamed, engorged with blood, or strangulated (see Section 65).

If the diarrhea is slight yet prolonged and does not respond to simple remedies, it may be just one symptom of some other, generalized disease. Don't treat yourself too long.

8. Effects of Diarrhea

On April 13, 1919, in Amritsar, India, British troops fired on an unarmed crowd, killing 400 people. To draw world attention to the killings the father of nonviolent protest, the Mahatma (Great Soul) Mohandas Karamchand Gandhi started his most famous and most effective hunger strike. His self-sacrifice was eminently successful. He survived months of starvation and eventually saw the triumph of his ideas.

On November 19, 1972, Sean McStioffain, chief of staff of the Provisional Irish Republican Army, was imprisoned by the Irish government. He too went on a hunger strike, but in order to make his protest more effective, he decided to take neither food nor drink. His condition deteriorated rapidly, became grave in a matter of days. He was at death's door within a week, then consented to take some food and drink.

The difference between the reactions of the bodies of the two activists was that the one continued to take the stuff from which all life on this earth has sprung; the other did not. That stuff, the basic constituent of the primordial ooze, is water. Without it there is no life. Man can live for long periods without food. Some of my overweight patients could make it happily for six months. But without a steady supply of water, or while suffering a continued loss of water in excess of intake, life ends. This is one reason why diarrhea is potentially so very serious.

Another reason why diarrhea can be so serious is that, with the water and nutrients, down the plumbing also go vitally important minerals and salts—especially potassium salts. Lack of potassium salts in the body has the effect of making you tired and listless and weak. Potassium is necessary for the smooth functioning of all muscles. In extreme potassium lack the heart muscle itself can stop functioning.

Potassium, sodium, and certain other salts are chemically classed as electrolytes: when they are dissolved in water, they release atoms—called ions—which are capable of carrying electric charges. All electrolytes are either acids or alkalies. Intestinal contents lost in diarrhea are alkaline. Loss of alkali results in acidosis. If there is also vomiting, as in the common illness called gastroenteritis—then acid stomach contents are lost as well. This may result in the swinging back of the body's acid-alkali balance toward normal—but at the expense of a quantitative loss of the acid. If vomiting is the predominant factor, as in some forms of food poisoning, then the clinical state may be that of an alkalosis.

Thus, severe diarrhea gives trouble on three fronts: through the loss of water, the loss of potassium, and the disturbance of the body's acid-base balance. (Base is another name for alkali.) Under this combined onslaught, life can be subdued very quickly. Whereas Sean McStioffain survived for ten or twelve days when not taking water or any other nourishment, a severe continuous diarrhea-producing illness, such as acute bacillary dysentery or cholera, can kill a patient in two days. True, in the case of these scourges there are other factors operating against the individual, such as the toxicity of the bacteria themselves. But the cause of death is water depletion, called dehydration, the loss of potassium and of some other electrolytes, and acid-alkali imbalance. Prevent or correct these and the patient will live.

It follows that the cornerstone of treatment of all cases and varieties of diarrhea is first the restoration of lost water. If the diarrhea bout proves mild—as is usually the case in summer diarrheas or overeating diarrheas—then the body can be expected to look after the regulation of the acid-alkali balance itself. Also, the body possesses huge stores of potassium and is quite able to mobilize these whenever the need arises. If there is little or no vomiting, the best way to take water is by mouth. One should, however, stop eating. Any food taken by mouth is liable to cause vomiting, as well as go through the stomach and intestines at such a speed that it is not likely to provide the body with much nourishment.

If there is significant vomiting or if the patient for some reason cannot swallow water or if the loss of water from the bowels is extreme or if there is significant loss of potassium and alkali, then the water with the needed electrolytes must be given directly into the bloodstream by infusion into a vein.

For detailed instructions on the home treatment of various types of diarrhea see Section 19.

9. Diarrhea in Babies

The gurgling, cooing, squealing, wet at both ends, soft, cuddly, and delightful creature that is humanity at birth is extremely vulnerable to dehydration. And no wonder. At a birth weight of seven pounds, the lack or loss of 2 ounces of water is equivalent to a lack or loss of almost 2 quarts of water in the case of a 170-pound adult. The newborn infant who is yelling lustily in the morning can develop a gastroenteritis or other severe form of diarrhea and be ready for a shoebox-size casket in the evening. Luckily for him or her, and luckily for the survival of the human race, this kind of extremely explosive diarrhea is rare, for several reasons. One is that the newborn receives the gift of certain antibodies and much resistance to various bacteria from his mother. That resistance is unfortunately short-lived. Most of it is dissipated after the first few weeks of life, but at the beginning of independent existence, it is vital. Additional bacterial antibodies are fed to children by mothers who breast-feed their babies. This is especially important in underdeveloped nations, where standards of hygiene are low. In North America the domestic water supply is reliably pure. Public Health authorities see to this. Cows' milk, the basis of almost all formulas, is sold pasteurized and is processed and transported in sterilized containers. Standards of home cleanliness are generally high.

Nevertheless, cases of explosive, extremely severe

infectious gastroenteritis of infants still occur, especially in children who are fed formulas.

Bottle-fed babies are also prone to develop various forms of less severe diarrhea. (More about this later in Sections 12–14.) The reason for this is that, in addition to the lack of milk-contained maternal antibodies, formula-fed babies receive a less than perfect substitute. Only human milk is by nature exactly tailored to the requirements of human infants. Cows' milk, on the other hand, is perfect for calves. Human milk is not drawn off by a milking machine that goes on the blink at times. It is not piped through hoses that someone may have forgotten to clean sometime. It is not pooled in huge storage tanks. It is not transported hundreds of miles and is not passed through bottling machines fitted with nozzles and taps and valves and valve washers that are difficult to keep sterile at the best of dairies. It is not jolted in the milkman's van and is not left standing in the dust outside your door or in a store. Nor is it spray-dried, powdered, generally messed with; it does not need to be reconstituted, with no slips in your own sterile formula-preparation technic, before use. Breast milk on the other hand goes directly from producer to consumer.

10. Acute Infectious Diarrhea of the Infant or Child

As was noted in Section 9, explosive, life-endangering diarrheas do not often occur in places such as Canada, the United States, and the countries of Western Europe. Such diseases are not unknown there: most practicing doctors see a case or two every few months, and there are pediatricians, Public Health officers, and infectious-diseases specialists who earn their livelihood from the treatment of just such problems. It is to the credit of these doctors that large-scale epidemics of explosive diarrheas of infants are almost unheard of and that individual cases are treated efficiently and not allowed to progress to critical stages.

The specific diseases that cause explosive diarrheas are more fully described in the sections dealing with gastroenteritis (19), influenzal enteritis (20), staphylococcal and other types of food poisoning (21), and the enteric pestilences (22). Treatment of these diseases is properly the province of specialists. What is important is that every mother be able to recognize when her child's simple diarrhea shades into seriousness, when she should give up on home remedies and promptly seek medical help.

Babies and children suffer from diarrhea very frequently indeed. On most occasions there is no need to drop everything and run to a doctor or a hospital because baby's stools are a little loose. Most by far of these simple diarrheas are due to feeding problems. They are described and their treatment is given in Sections 11 and 13. Some are due to milk allergies (see Section 14), and some others are due to other causes.

Once the normal infant has expelled the black meconium from his or her intestinal tract (see Section 3), he or she soon settles down with regular passages of golden-yellow, nonsmelling, salvelike stools; the average frequency of evacuation is one to two stools per day for the formula-fed baby and two to four stools per day for the breast-fed baby. There are also perfectly healthy infants who pass motions only once per day or more rarely only once every two to three days. Suspect the onset of nutritional diarrhea if that regularity is either never attained or first attained, then upset. Suspect the onset of infectious diarrhea if that number of daily stools doubles and the child looks and acts ill.

If your baby suddenly produces six or eight or ten stools during one day—say, a stool every two to three hours—should you worry? The answer is no. Should you take notice, count the number of stools, look carefully at them, watch for other symptoms, try to figure out why the change has occurred? The answer is definitely yes. If in spite of the looseness of the stools your baby still smiles at you, still coos and gurgles happily, still sleeps at most of the usual times and yells a bit in between, then there is obviously nothing much to worry about—yet. Chances are that your baby is suffering from a minor degree of nutritional imbalance (see Sections 11–13).

However, let us assume that this looseness either persists at the same rate of a stool every two to three hours for a whole day or longer, or else that the frequency of the motions increases and there is a stool almost every hour. This is obviously more than just a passing looseness of the bowels. This now is diarrhea. With it your infant becomes listless, either sleeps or dozes most of the time, looks pale and unhappy when awake, and becomes irritable, that is, cries and struggles when handled or disturbed. Let us further assume that you have taken your child's temperature and find it either normal or only slightly elevated or slightly subnormal. Should you worry? The answer is still no. Should you become concerned? The answer is yes. This may be just a slightly more severe form of nutritional disturbance. It may, however, be the beginning of something more serious. Babies and children get sick quickly—bouncing around in the morning and laid out flat in the afternoon. Thank goodness they also recover quickly—they may be full of life and mischief again by evening. With these symptoms you should definitely adopt the measures of giving no food whatever but instead frequently administering, in small sips, boiled cooled water with a little sugar added, as described fully in Section 19.

Now let us assume that your baby continues to pass a semiliquid or liquid stool every hour and that the stools are green. The dietary measures alone have not worked. Now is the time to use a nonprescription type of diarrhea remedy such as Kaopectate (made by Upjohn), given in ample doses either every one or two hours or after the passage of every loose stool. This—together with the dietary measures of no food, sugared boiled, cooled water given very frequently but only in small sips—will probably stop all simple and most moderate infectious diarrheas. But for the sake of argument let us assume that it did not. The green stools continue. The odd color indicates that intestinal contents are now rushing through your child's intestinal tract at great speed. The color comes from bile that has not had time to change from its original green to yellow or gold or orange-brown in the short time it was whisked through the length of the intestine. Let us assume further that your baby's irritability has increased. He now whimpers or cries almost continuously, and neither letting him rest in the crib nor walking the floor with him in your arms seems to do much good. He is by now not only pale but pale gray. There are rings around the eyes. The nose is pale white and pinched.

The lips are thin. The hands and fingers are no longer normal pink but are white. As he cries, the cry is louder and more pitiful every so often and with that extra yelp he draws his knees up to his chest. Some of the boiled, cooled sugared water and some of the medicine you have given him is vomited. Most of it is refused. Should you now worry? Definitely yes.

This is a more serious stage of diarrhea, which now merits the name "enteritis." If the vomiting increases or if the infant now also vomits spontaneously—that is, not only brings up the fluids and medicine you have just given him but also retches up acid-smelling stomach mucus—then the illness is a gastroenteritis.

The severity of a given case of gastroenteritis depends entirely on the length of time that elapses between its onset and the start of efficient treatment. By this I mean treatment in a hospital, with proper laboratory determination of the exact degree of dehydration and the exact definition of the acid-base imbalance that must be corrected. Intravenous fluids are the cornerstone of the treatment of these cases. Since an infant is so small, the calculation and administration of just the right fluid replacements call for the skill of experts. With symptoms such as these, there is little time to be lost. Take your baby to the hospital without delay.

Let us finally assume that for some reason medical help was not available in time and that your baby is still more sick. The stools are now not only green but are tinged with blood. In extreme cases they may be completely bloody. This means that the inflammation of the lining of the intestine is so severe that it oozes blood. The irritability has given way to exhaustion, with apathy, immobility, and stupor. The baby can be roused with difficulty, or perhaps cannot be roused at all. The whole body is limp: when you try to raise the child, the head sags back and the arms and legs trail behind the trunk as if on a badly stuffed doll. The skin color is no longer pale gray but is deathly white in the case of a white child or dull charcoal gray in the case of a black child. The baby feels cold to the touch. The eyes are deeply sunken in their sockets. The cheekbones are prominent, as if there were no flesh at all between bones and skin. The thin lips are drained of color. The breath comes in short, infrequent gasps. The pulsebeat is almost imperceptible. The trunk and the bloated belly are still racked by spasms, but the baby now no longer has the strength to draw up his knees.

This is a stage of gastroenteritis, in which even the best, most efficient treatment may fail. Life is about to depart from the wretched little body.

Don't let the disease go that far.

11. Overfeeding Diarrhea of the Infant or Child

Milk, especially cows' milk, is potent stuff. The human infant who at his first weigh-in tips the scales at around seven pounds will, on a diet of nothing but milk, double his birthweight in four and a half months and will triple his birthweight in twelve months. Naturally this rate of growth must then slow down, or the infant would grow up to be a whale.

Doting mothers and grandmothers do not understand this. They like to see their baby keep on eating. They persist in feeding the chubby little thing full cream milk, which—homogenized or not—contains over 5 percent butterfat. To them human milk looks bluish and "weak"; 2 percent dairy milk seems not good enough either. They add cereal mixes to the formula earlier than such additions are recommended.

Because babies are generally tough—they will digest

and thrive on almost anything out of a bottle or can that is white and has originated in a cow's udder or on a farmer's field—the result is that far too many of them are overfat. In the process of getting overweight many of the little tummies naturally rebel. It happens that the infants' intestines know better than their well-meaning mothers. The result is diarrhea.

If the overfeeding is done routinely, then this diarrhea is likely habitual and low grade. In this case the normal daily number of evacuations is increased but slightly, though it may double. If the overfeeding is occasional, actual bouts of diarrhea occur. You can tell what is happening simply by looking at the stools.

From too much fat in the formula the stools are bulky and actually look greasy. There is a fatty, greasy stain on the diaper. Often these stools smell. When they are disposed of into the toilet, they do not sink but float on top of the water.

The treatment here is obvious. Cut down on the amount of fat in the formula. Switch to 2 percent milk or to a powdered preparation and reconstitute it with water exactly according to the directions on the can; if anything, add a little more water than the directions call for. Do not again yield to the temptation of making the mixture just a little richer than the instructions call for, "just to make sure he gets enough to eat and grows up big and strong." If you do, you will be causing trouble again.

From too much starch and sugar in the formula the stools become frothy from fermentation. They look like pancake batter that has been churned in an electric mixer or blender at too fast a speed. They smell sour.

Again the treatment is obvious. Cut down on the carbohydrate overfeeding by adding less sugar or syrup or molasses, or else switch to a powdered preparation that contains less carbohydrate.

Note that the amounts of carbohydrate, fat, water, and protein contained in formula preparations are always clearly marked on the label.

Generally speaking, in all feeding problems of infants it is always better to first vary the amount of water added to the formula than to switch to a different preparation, because after you have fed your child one formula for a while you know how she or he reacts to it. You have experience with that particular brand. Adding a little more or a little less water to it from day to day, depending on circumstances and responses, is in the nature of making fine adjustments. If you switch to something else every time there is a slight feeding difficulty, you must every time learn how your baby reacts to the different mix.

12. Underfeeding Diarrhea of the Infant or Child

Underfeeding results in diarrhea in that the stools are liquid or nearly so and are greenish or brownish-green from bile that has not had enough food to act upon in the intestinal tract. The normal bile color comes through unchanged. Depending on whether there is or is not a sufficient intake of water, the thin greenish stools are or are not frequent.

The commonest cause of underfeeding is not neglect or cruelty on the part of the mother. The usual reason is that the holes in the nipple of the formula bottle are too small and do not allow a free flow. The baby sucks and strains and gulps and swallows air and gets collicky pains from all that swallowed air—and goes hungry. In between, the desperate mother gives the infant some glucose or sugar water, which he or she drinks greedily.

The water alone goes through the small nipple holes easier than the thick formula, so the child temporarily at least gets a full stomach and thankfully does not develop dehydration.

Paradoxically, a nipple with holes too big can cause underfeeding too: The child sucks on the nipple and gets a big mouthful and noseful of formula. He or she chokes, spits, coughs, swallows air, and becomes afraid that the next mouthful will produce the same result. So, being much more clever than his mother gives him credit for, he starts the next sucking action very carefully indeed. But once more there comes a big stream, just like the Chinese water torture. So he refuses to try again and becomes confused, fussy, irritable, gassy, and collicky, and, in spite of mother's best efforts, he remains hungry. Poor mother then remembers seeing some advertisement for gripe water or other sedative. That quietens the infant up to a point. But the child is not healthy, he or she does not gain weight, his or her appearance shows that something is wrong, and a look at the stools tells the story.

The treatment of these disturbances is laughably easy. Experiment with different nipples and different-size nipple holes. You can always make the nipple holes larger by passing through them a red hot pin or needle, which you hold with a pair of pliers while you heat it on your kitchen stove. Just be sure to rub off any bits of melted or burned rubber from around the enlarged nipple holes before you sterilize the nipple for feeding. If the nipple holes are too big, then you just have to buy another nipple.

13. Diarrhea Due to Wrong Formula

Diarrhea, together with failure to thrive, can result from using a formula that is not right for your baby. This sort of thing is popularly called allergy, but allergy really means something else. Many commercial preparations today are made up of weird mixtures of vegetable products such as oleo oil, corn oil, soybeans, various chemical stabilizers, conditioners, thickness and freshness preservers, and other additives besides basic skimmed cows' milk and a variety of synthetic vitamins and minerals. The cows from which some of that milk has come may have been receiving antibiotics in their fodder. The vegetables from which the oils are extracted have been grown with the help of fertilizers and insecticides. These concoctions are then homogenized, evaporated, pasteurized or sterilized, canned, and finally fancy-packaged for your visual approval.

I have no intention of knocking these brews . . . too much. They are perfectly suitable for most babies. Healthy infants are surprisingly strong individuals with brand-new, unused, unmaltreated, healthy digestions. They will digest and thrive on almost anything. But your baby is not in the category of "most average babies." He or she is an individual quite unique in all the world, and the cocktails that are excellent for others might not be right for him. The result may again be diarrhea, or it may be some other disturbance.

As was mentioned in Section 11 and contrary to

what may be inferred from the above, the treatment of mild diarrhea in such cases is not to switch to a different formula right away. You cannot be sure that some constituent in the mix you are using is responsible for the disturbance. Every time you switch brands you first have to experiment a bit to find the right concentration and the right feeding frequency. Your baby may not necessarily be better off. The right thing to do is first to change the nipple, next to change the bottle, and next to make sure that all bottles and nipples and utensils are truly clean and sterilized before each feeding. Next try slightly different dilutions—add more water or add less water to the formula and be sure that the water has been boiled or otherwise sterilized and properly cooled. Make sure that the formula is the proper temperature. Only after you have tried all that should you change the formula brand.

14. True Intestinal Allergy

In true intestinal allergy the stools are wet, yellow, bulky, gassy, and mixed with mucus. Some evacuations may consist mostly of mucus and the mucus may be tinged with bright red blood.

Mucus is the surface lubricant of mucous membranes, such as the linings of the nasal passages and the lining of the whole of the intestine from the stomach onward. It is normally a clear, thick, slimy fluid that serves as a flypaper-type trap against dust in the respiratory passages and as a lubricant in the intestinal passages.

Just as in respiratory allergy the increase in nasal secretions result in a running nose, so in intestinal allergy the amounts of mucus secreted are also increased. With normal stools the amount of mucus passed is so small that you do not notice it in the toilet bowl. In true allergy it is there to see, and if the allergy is severe, blood is passed with it.

The passage of bulky, yellow, wet, mucoid diarrhea is not the only symptom of intestinal allergy. With it the child also suffers from nausea, vomiting, tummy pains, and cramps. In typical cases the feeding pattern tells as much as the appearance of the stools. The infant yells with hunger. He is given a bottle of formula. He takes a gulp or two, then seems not to like the taste and refuses to take more. In a minute or so he again yells with hunger, is offered the same food again, and once more finds it not to his taste. Eventually he seems to think better of it and takes the rest of the bottle. Then he vomits it all up. Then he is hungry again, yet unhappy about further feeds, irritable, and cranky. He cries with colic and passes much gas.

A look at the stools gives the answer. Another look, this time at his buttocks, confirms it. These babies get the most horrible diaper rashes, with the worst of the irritation centered not about the urinary passages but about the anus.

If this sort of thing is happening to your baby and if the baby is on cows' milk, then switch to one of the vegetable-product formulas, usually to one based on soybeans. If, on the other hand, your baby is on a compound formula now, then switch to two percent cows' milk with a little sugar or syrup added (about a teaspoon to each six ounces). If the symptoms are very severe or prolonged, see a doctor.

Intestinal allergies are not lifelong afflictions. Babies usually get over mild or simple problems of this sort in a matter of a few months, without any special treatment. They may subsequently develop some other allergic problems such as eczema. In the majority of cases, the illness is not serious and does not lead to anything serious.

15. Intussusception

Intussusception is a condition peculiar to babies from about three to twenty-four months of age, in which a portion of the intestine infolds into itself like a telescope. When fully developed, the involved part of the intestine looks like the sleeve of a long-sleeved sweater that has been partially turned inside out, so that in one area there is a triple thickness of sleeve material infolded into itself and out again. It develops in otherwise and previously healthy, husky babies with a frightening rapidity. The bright, alert, and contented infant is suddenly seized with severe tummy pain, cries, draws up his knees to his chin, frequently vomits, and passes first a bit of normal stool, then typically some thin and watery stool, and finally a blood-stained, congealing, mucoid excretion that looks like red currant jelly.

The preliminary thin watery stool may be absent. Passage of the red currant jelly may also be absent but if present is absolutely diagnostic. Watch for it at any time from two to twelve hours after the onset of any bout of an acute tummy pain. There may not be much of this jelly. Even a teaspoon, even just a smear of it on the diaper, is significant.

Intussusception is not a common disease, but it occurs often enough that parents should be aware that it exists. It is a dangerous condition requiring emergency treatment. That treatment can sometimes consist of an enema on an x-ray table where the pressure of the enema fluid is used by a radiologist to push the infolding out of itself. More often an emergency operation is necessary. To be successful the operation must be performed early, before the infolded portion of the gut becomes inflamed and swollen and ruptures, and before generalized peritonitis supervenes.

Never give any laxative to a child suffering from an acute tummy ache. If you think that the cause may be constipation, then the use of a glycerine suppository once is permissible. If that does not work, call your doctor. Intussusception is just one disease that can be made terribly worse by laxatives. There are others—appendicitis, for instance. Laxatives have no place at all in the treatment of any abdominal pain in the child or in an adult.

16. Celiac Disease of the Infant or Child (Malabsorption Syndrome)

The word "celiac" is derived from ancient Greek and means "abdominal." The phrase "malabsorption syndrome" means that this is not a well-defined and understood illness but rather an assortment of symptoms that are caused by deficient absorption of food nutrients. The child who suffers from it may be getting the best and most nutritious diet in the world, but some ingredients of the diet just go through his stomach and intestines and out in the stools, unabsorbed. The net effect in severe cases is that the child is malnourished and undernourished. He not only suffers from diarrhea but does not gain weight, does not develop properly. I personally call really bad cases the heartbreak diarrhea disease.

Luckily the very severe varieties of this illness are quite rare. Luckily again, a tremendous amount of research is being undertaken to unravel the extremely complicated biochemical changes that characterize it. This research is expensive. Public appeals for funds by the Cystic Fibrosis Foundation and by other similar societies merit your support. Their efforts have already borne considerable fruit: the awe and mystery and terror that once characterized celiac disease are no more. It is already recognized that there are thirty-odd varieties and subgroups of it. Efficient treatment for some of the varieties already exists. More will follow.

The feature that all varieties of celiac disease have in common is steatorrhea: the passage of undigested fat in the stools. The evacuations not only are frequent and loose but are bulky and greasy and have a foul odor. As noted in Section 4, the passage of greasy, foul-smelling stools that float on the water in the toilet bowl occurs occasionally in babies (also in adults) whose recent diet contained too much fat. In celiac disease it is the fats and sometimes also the starches contained in balanced diets that are not absorbed.

The thirty-odd varieties of celiac disease can be roughly divided into four groups:

1. True celiac disease (fat and wheat gluten intolerance)
2. Infantile steatorrhea (fat intolerance)
3. Starch and sugar intolerance
4. Cystic fibrosis disease (fat *and* starch intolerance)

In the first two main groups of celiac disease the inability of the child's digestion to deal with fats is by far the predominant problem. In starch and sugar intolerance the stools are unmistakably bubbly and frothy from excessive fermentation of the undigested carbohydrates by intestinal bacteria. Cystic fibrosis is the most disabling. Unable to digest either fats or starches, the child has difficulties with most ordinary, staple, everyday foods. As if this were not enough, there is an additional problem: These children also suffer from a defective and deficient production of mucus in the respiratory passages and in the lungs, which leads to bouts of bronchitis and pneumonia and to the formation of lung abscesses. Accompanying it all, there is a marked retardation of growth. Diarrhea in cystic fibrosis not only is chronic but is punctuated by acute, explosive bouts, called crises.

The first symptoms of most varieties of celiac disease occur at birth but in less severe cases may be delayed until the age of three or six months. Starch intolerance may not show up until the child is five years old.

The treatment of these conditions is very specialized. It centers on the devising of diets that the patients' digestions can deal with. The diets must be tasty and satisfying or they will refuse them, yet the diets must also be balanced to supply the nutrients that the growing bodies need so desperately.

In cystic fibrosis, in addition to attention to diet problems, treatment of lung complications must at times take place in special chambers or tents in which the air is saturated with mucus-dissolving chemicals—definitely a task for experts only.

17. Nervous Diarrhea

Have you heard stories of a sudden uncontrolled diarrhea afflicting a student at an important examination or a soldier during a bombardment? The stories can be made to sound funny—but only if the trouble involves someone else. Nervous diarrhea is no joke.

It can happen to anybody. Toddlers and small children suffer from it. Teenagers and "tough" young guys are not immune. Adults and older people get it, too. Naturally it leads to embarrassment and worse—and to fear that it may happen again. If it does recur a few times, especially in the case of a child, the result may well be that the trifle shy individual becomes increasingly nervous, introspective, and even disturbed. He may in later life shun all excitement, strive to avoid confrontations, and become unfit for challenging jobs. It can become a real disability.

Let us assume that you are the parent of a toddler or grade schooler who does suffer from this kind of thing. What can you do?

First, sit down and analyze the kind of experiences that have resulted in his suffering from nervous diarrhea. Recall—write it down, preferably—especially all the occasions when the diarrhea proved so severe and so explosive that your child did not have time to get to the bathroom but actually filled his pants.

You will probably come up with stories of emotional upsets. Some of them may have been painful for you, too. Some of them may have been major crises—a death in the family, for instance, or a big row between yourself and your spouse. The child's diarrhea at that time was likely either immediate or was delayed by a day or a week. A major crisis or catastrophe may have caused a lengthy period of loss of control of his bowels, then.

But perhaps at other times you cannot recall any big upset that preceded the incontinence. Were there any minor crises that your child may have felt deeply? Was there unhappiness in the home? Were you unduly preoccupied with something else, or with somebody else? Children have their own feelings, many of which are centered on their continuing to experience a sense of security, of being wanted, of being loved. I have come across instances of nervous diarrhea that started when the family moved to a different city or even when the child only had to change schools. The parents were busy with the hundreds of details involved in making the move. Nobody thought of explaining the changes to the child.

If your child is prone to this sort of thing and if an upset of daily routine is unavoidable, then by all means see your doctor and request a gentle sedative to help him over the hurdle. But remember that the medicine or the tablet by itself will not be sufficient. You will still have to spend time to comfort and to love. Do not punish your child for the "accident." Tell him that you do not approve, but do not make an undue fuss about it. Clean him up gently; small children have a peculiar psychologic idea that their bowel movements are their "own" property and do not particularly like to have their possession roughly taken away from them. Never, never ridicule the older child about it.

What if you are an adult and you yourself have this problem? What should you do?

First, sit down and write down and analyze all previous occasions when nervous diarrhea has hit you. Spend considerable time on this. Were your fears, your nervousness, your tension justified by the severity or the intensity of the stimulus or the occasion that prompted it? Could you face a similar occasion or similar emergency now without diarrhea? After all, it happened to you before. The sky did not fall down. You now have experience of that particular disaster and of that other one, too, and you know now that neither of them proved as bad as you had perhaps feared. Think of it: by having gone through it before, you are now expert in dealing with it. Consequently it will not affect you like that again.

Second, if your analysis shows that there is more than nervousness to this, then read the section that deals with the irritable colon syndrome (Section 48). The answers to your problems are probably there. If not and if you are afraid that some forthcoming event will prove embarrassing to you in this manner, then also see your doctor. Explain your difficulty to him. He should be able to prescribe a sedative for you that you should need to take only very occasionally. Or else your doctor may suggest some psychotherapy or may advise you to undergo a course of hypnosis. You can be cured.

18. Acute Dietary Diarrhea

"Johnny stole the neighbor's apples—now Johnny is sick with the runs." So goes the tale of one of nature's educational knocks. Nature is a hard taskmaster. It does not believe that corporal punishment is either undemocratic or demeaning. Stick your hand into a fire. The lesson you'll learn is administered immediately. The punishment for your ignorance is instantaneous. The rehabilitation will be painful. The guarantee that you will not transgress again is gilt-edged.

In Johnny's case the lesson was that unripe apples have a laxating effect and that the degree of laxation produced is roughly proportional to the amount of laxative taken. It is up to his parents and teachers to tell him that other fruits and vegetables have similar effects and that yet other vegetable substances have it in a potency that makes them poisons if ingested inadvertently or valued drugs if taken in the right circumstances and amounts.

Practically all fresh fruits have a laxative effect, especially if unripe, be they apples or pears or grapes or plums or berries or citrus. They act through a combination of specific chemicals and their soft yet undigestible bulk or roughage. A balanced diet should always include fresh fruit and fresh vegetable produce. The accent is on freshness and tenderness. Ripe or processed vegetables generally lose their laxative potencies. There are exceptions—notably prunes and dried figs—which must be either steeped in water or boiled in order to regain this attribute. Overripe and dried produce such as peas, beans, corn, oranges, and raisins do not have that effect.

The purely medicinal lesson is obvious. If one suffers from diarrhea, then fresh fruit and produce should be temporarily avoided. If one suffers from constipation, then the intake of fresh fruit and fresh tender produce should be increased.

The treatment of acute dietary diarrhea is first to get on with it. The sooner the offending irritant is out of your system and on its way down the sewage pipes in the direction of the sanitation works, the better. Since your intestines are now overactive and inflamed, the less additional foodstuff they have to deal with, the better. Chances are that anything else you now eat will also go through you very quickly, and you will get very little or no nutrition. So eat nothing. This will grant your gut a period of time for recuperation and rest. A general principle in medicine is that an inflamed part of the body needs rest. A sprained ankle or a twisted knee improves quickest if the patient stays off his feet. An upset digestion recovers best if it does not have work to perform.

You must, however, drink. Your body needs a constant supply of water. The water is best taken slightly warmed, in small sips, frequently. You may add a little sugar, which will keep your energy up and prevent you from feeling faint. Do not take fruit juices.

Once your diarrhea is slightly better, switch to weak tea with sugar added. Tea contains tannin, which has an astringent, sedative effect on the inflamed intestinal lining. Once you feel better still, eat the kind of food you would normally feed to a small baby—rice or barley or wheat cereal cooked with water, then with milk, with sugar added. If you can take that, you are obviously on your way to recovery and can resume taking a more normal diet, but still without irritants: avoid fried foods and spicy foods, and definitely leave out fresh fruits until you feel quite well again.

In acute dietary diarrhea, medicines are generally not needed. Save your money; the graduated diet outlined above will get you over your bout quicker than drugs would do it. If, however, your diarrhea should be so severe that it degenerates into a bout of enteritis, then drugs will be necessary. (See Section 19 for details.)

19. Gastroenteritis

Next to nutritional or dietary bowel disturbances, the commonest cause of diarrhea and vomiting in infants, children, and adults is inflammation of the intestinal tract. The expression "gastroenteritis" means inflammation of the stomach and of the intestines. When inflammation of the stomach predominates, the main symptom is vomiting and the condition is called gastritis. When inflammation of the intestines is the main problem, the main disturbance is diarrhea and the condition is called enteritis. Usually the two coexist. One usually comes before the other. When the inflammation is clearing, vomiting subsides first; diarrhea lasts a little longer.

The term "inflammation" describes the changes that living tissue undergoes when it is subjected to an injury. It is a defense reaction and consists of two parts. The object of the first part is to destroy and remove the irritant. The object of the second part is to repair the damage. It is a fascinating process that has engrossed men of science for 2,000 years. We have to go back to Celsus in the first century A.D. for the description of the "cardinal signs" of inflammation: rubor, tumor, calor, and dolor, in words that every student of medicine still learns today: "Now the characteristics of inflammation are four: redness and swelling, with heat and pain."

Gastroenteritis is a large group of diseases, all of which manifest more-or-less similar symptoms: vomiting and diarrhea. They differ in speed of onset, duration, and severity. Their causes can be divided into the following:

1. Influenzal—due to viruses
2. Bacterial—due to various bacteria
3. Chemical—due to chemicals, alcohol, and poisons
4. Allergic—due to an exaggerated body reaction to otherwise harmless substances.

This section deals with the symptoms and treatment common to all kinds of gastroenteritis. Certain particular kinds are described further in succeeding sections on influenzal enteritis (20), food poisoning (21), the enteric pestilences (22), and alcohol, drugs, and poisons (23).
fants are particularly susceptible. Every child goes through a bout of it at least once in his young life. Home treatment of the common-sense variety cures

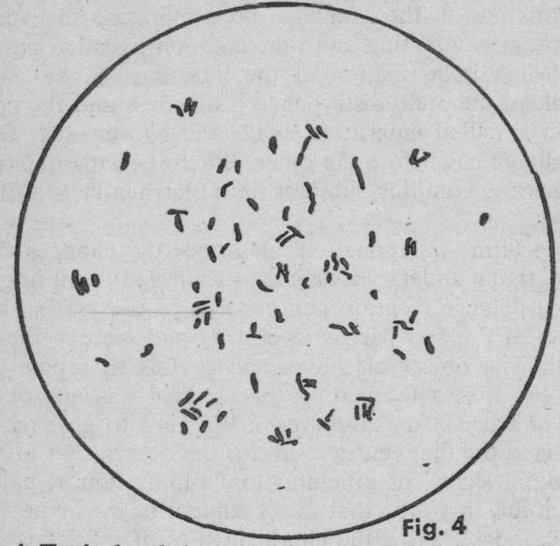

Fig. 4. Typical rod shaped bacteria. There are thousands of varieties. These could be colon bacteria (B. coli), or typhoid bacteria (Salmonella typhi), or one of the organisms that cause dysentery (e.g. Shigella), or a harmless variety. Bacteriologists tell them apart by staining them different colors, or by growing them under different culture conditions.

most cases, but there are times when admission to a hospital and intravenous fluids are the only hope. Unfortunately, there are also times when even the best treatment fails. Severe gastroenteritis is a potential killer.

The treatment of mild gastroenteritis is exactly the same as that of dietary diarrhea, described in the preceding section (18). Drugs are not necessary.

In more severe cases, especially when inflammation of the stomach is a large factor (gastritis), the stomach lining becomes so inflamed that it may not be able to deal with water. The thing to do then is to drink the water in very, very tiny sips every few minutes. This may do the trick. If even tiny sips result in retching, then try a mixture of bicarbonate of soda, available in most households as baking soda (not baking powder—that is something else). Mix a heaping teaspoon of baking soda into a glass (eight ounces) of lukewarm water. Take a tiny sip of this mixture every ten to fifteen minutes—make that glass of bicarbonate solution last several hours. With a bit of luck this will settle your stomach sufficiently so that you can take sugared water or sugared tea next.

If diarrhea is the predominant complaint and if the treatment outlined above is not sufficient, then the household remedy is to try bicarbonate of soda solution taken in somewhat larger doses, alternating with spoonfuls of powdered skim milk batter. To prepare the latter, take a large cup of powdered skimmed milk. Add water a little at a time, while stirring continuously. To be just right it should be of the consistency of pancake batter.

Caution! Do not treat your gastritis or gastroenteritis with bicarbonate of soda in larger doses than those mentioned above, and in no case for longer than twenty-four hours, or else electrolyte problems will occur. The stomach contents that you are vomiting are acid. The bicarbonate is alkaline. Too much alkali will result in your developing the complication of alkalosis.

Caution again! Skim milk batter is not to everybody's taste. Try it, but if the taste makes you even more nauseated, then do not persevere with it.

If this still does not work, then go out and buy one of the following:

Activated charcoal (many manufacturers)
Atasorb (Lilly)
Kalpec Wyeth)
Kao-Con (Upjohn)
Kaopectate (Upjohn)

All of the above are available without prescription. All are suitable for both children and adults. Except for charcoal, which is an adsorbent, all contain kaolin (a purified clay) and pectin. None are poisonous. Allergies to them may possibly occur but are rare. They should be taken in full doses as detailed on their labels and always together with the water and dietary regimens outlined above. They will effectively control 95 percent of all gastroenteritis cases.

Let us now assume that you are very unfortunate and that you are having a very severe bout of gastroenteritis. Neither the sugar water nor the bicarbonate and skimmed milk nor the above drugs work for you. What should you do?

The drugs to try next may be available where you live without a prescription. Chances are that they are not. All contain mixtures of kaolin and pectin, but with either antibiotics and/or intestinal sedatives added. Many of the intestinal sedatives are classified as narcotics. You will have to consult a doctor, who will probably prescribe one of the following:

Cremomycin (MSD)
Cremosuccidine (MSD)
Donnagel (Robins)
Donnagel P.G. (Robins)
Donnagel with Neomycin (Robins)
Kaomycin (Upjohn)
Parelixir (Purdue Frederick)

Parpectolin (Rorer)
Pomalin (Winthrop; may not be available in U.S.)

If these still do not cure you, then you will have to be admitted to a hospital. You will require treatment with intravenous fluids as well as other medications. If you have not delayed seeking medical attention too long, your chances of recovery are excellent.

Once you are in the hospital your doctor will investigate the exact bacterial or other cause of your disease. It may be that you are not suffering from gastroenteritis but from one of the other vomiting and diarrhea-producing diseases described elsewhere in this book.

20. Influenzal Enteritis—The "Stomach Flu"

The expression "stomach flu" is a double euphemism. Since it isn't "polite" to talk about one's bowels, the "stomach" part of the expression refers to them. The "flu" part means diarrhea. True, in influenzal enteritis there is almost always also a gastric (stomach) component, which shows up as vomiting; however, diarrhea is the predominant symptom. With it there is fever and a degree of debility that amounts to total prostration, which is the outstanding characteristic of this disease and which distinguishes it from other varieties of gastroenteritis. Most people have been through it at least once and can speak from personal experience. With the diarrhea there come muscular pains of the arms, legs, back, and head—everything hurts—and the weakness one feels is overpowering.

This type of gastroenteritis hits suddenly. It is contagious. It occurs in epidemics, but unlike staph food poisoning, typhoid, or cholera, the infection does not appear to spread by eating contaminated food or drinking infected water but by direct person-to-person contact. Is the cause of it a form of epidemic influenza?

Strange as this may sound, nobody is sure. Certainly doctors are aware of the disease epidemic influenza, which sweeps the world like a tidal wave every few years. In the years 1918–1919, just after World War I, it was responsible for over 22 million deaths. It hit so suddenly that people at work in the morning were dead in the afternoon. No pandemic so devastating has occurred ever before or since, but less severe waves have taken their toll in the nineteenth century and every three or four years since.

Epidemic and pandemic influenza is known to be a virus-caused disease that attacks predominantly the respiratory tract with initial symptoms of sneezing, dry cough, and congestion. It progresses to shortness of breath from a rapidly developing bronchitis and pneumonia, but with the same extreme weakness and prostration and the same muscular and joint and body pains that characterize influenzal enteritis. Its attack is similarly rapid. Its mode of spreading is by air transmission of droplets from coughs and sneezes. The transmission of epidemic enteritis is thought to be similar.

There are, however, important differences. Influenzal enteritis occurs in epidemics but to date thank goodness it has not struck in pandemic proportions. In fact, its epidemics are usually not at all widespread. Most important, it is not a killing disease. The vomiting, diarrhea, extreme weakness, and prostration usually all clear in a few days with little treatment.

This is one disease that regularly incurs the wrath of some doctors who should know better. It happens this way: The patient feels so ill and looks so ghastly that he or she or the relatives panic and demand that the doctor drop everything, interrupt his office hours, get out of his bed at 3:00 A.M., and see them. By the time the doctor gets around to examing the patient, the disease has quit. The patient and the relatives then try to explain just how bad things were a half-hour ago, while the doctor's blood pressure threatens to blow a blood vessel as he draws his own, very wrong conclusions about the state of his patient's psyche, about the "softness" of the generation that it is his misfortune to treat, and about his own harassed existence.

All this means that if you or your spouse or child suddenly suffer from abdominal cramps with initial vomiting, then with explosive diarrhea, and especially if all this comes together with an acute headache, with grinding pains in all the bones, with backache and a feeling of weakness and exhaustion so severe that even moving one arm is difficult and marching to the bathroom for yet another session on the throne almost impossible, do not think that the End is Nigh. It means that you have caught influenzal enteritis, otherwise known as the infamous stomach flu. It also means that you can look forward to a clearing of the illness as sudden as the onset was abrupt.

Beyond these symptoms, influenzal enteritis is a difficult ailment to diagnose scientifically. There are no quick or easy specific tests. Head and back pains, muscular pains, and the feeling of weakness are subjective symptoms, impossible to measure or grade. Some presumed cases are due to bacterial infections, food poisonings, accidental or otherwise ingestions of irritating chemicals in contaminated fruit or milk or water, short-lived allergies, nervous or hysterical diarrhea bouts, and so on.

There is no treatment that can be aimed against the cause of the trouble, the virus that is having a ball at your expense. Antibiotics do not work. Sulfa drugs are useless. Either or both may be prescribed by your doctor if he has doubts about the diagnosis, which will be the case especially if your bout continues longer than expected.

Influenzal enteritis is a variety of gastroenteritis. The symptomatic treatment outlined in Section 19 works well. It will be all that is needed in almost all cases.

One word of caution: The head pain, the back pains, the joint discomfort all tend to suggest to the unwary that perhaps the trouble is a cold or "rheumatism" with diarrhea added. Right away, then, one tends to remember TV advertisements for aspirin and assorted other quick pain relievers. Do not take any of these. Aspirin is a stomach irritant. When aspirin comes into contact with an already inflamed stomach lining it can start a hemorrhage. All the fast, fast pain relievers contain aspirin. Taking them will not help; it will make you feel even worse and can be downright dangerous.

21. Food Poisoning

In contrast to the vagueness of diagnosis in cases of influenzal enteritis (Section 20), there is no question in food poisoning. The villains are staphylococci, usually known as staph. Other bacteria have similar actions, and what is said here about staph applies to them too, but staph is the most important.

Staph are the most common bacteria found on the human body. They grow in clumps of little bells and are regularly found on everyone's skin. One of the many mysteries of life is why a person may harbor these germs for years and years without any trouble arising, and then one day the good neighbor relationship goes to pot. Staph are the germs responsible for pimples and spots and little infections about chewed fingernails and ingrowing toenails. For these we could forgive them. But they also cause boils and tonsillitis and abscesses. They are the bane of the surgeon and the terror of the operated-on patient because they infect operative wounds. They can invade a person's bloodstream and spread a plague of infection literally through every tissue of the body.

Staph are also responsible for food poisoning. Some strains of them are capable of producing a poison called a toxin. Moreover, they can do this while living outside the human body, feasting on such delicatessen as pastries and salads and fried chicken and custards and all manner of other prepared foods. How do they get mixed up with foods? From the hands of cooks, of course, whether the cook is mother or whether the cook is employed by a restaurant or a food processor. A colony of them may grow on just one side of a ham sandwich or on just one of a whole plate of tarts. If this

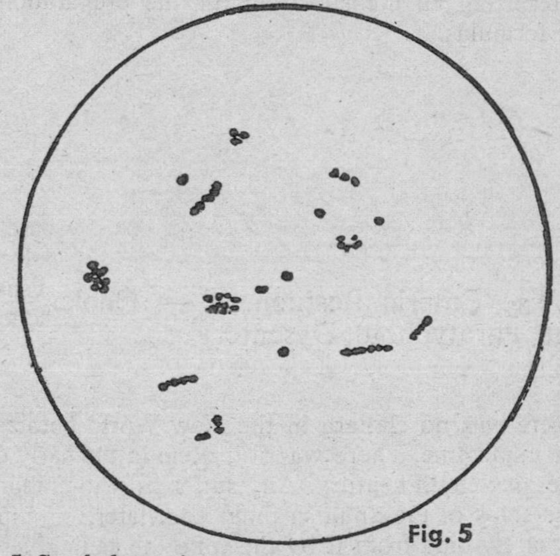

Fig. 5. Staphylococci grow in clumps of little balls.

happens, then the only person to get sick will be the one who happens to eat that particular slice of ham or that one cookie. It can be a sort of Russian roulette, played to the tune of "but he didn't eat anything different from the rest of us."

Quite often, however, everyone who has eaten the contaminated food gets sick. Then the cause is obvious.

To prevent staph food poisoning all hands preparing food must be free from any infection and clean. Cooking or boiling food that has been handled by contaminated hands is no salvation: the germs are killed by the heat, most of the toxins are not. Further, prepared foods must not be left standing, especially not left outside the refrigerator.

The bout of staph food poisoning itself is a typical attack of gastroenteritis. This is described and its treatment is given in Section 19. It is usually not dangerous to adults but can be very dangerous to children. The smaller the child, the greater the danger. The newborn baby is particularly susceptible—hence the emphasis on sterilizing all utensils used for the preparation of baby formulas.

22. The Enteric Pestilences — Cholera, Typhoid, Paratyphoid, Dysentery

There was no cholera in the New World before the white man came. There was still none in the early days of the nineteenth century. Any sufferers who embarked on the ships of the Spanish main and, later, on clipper ships surely died from it by the time the sailing vessels reached this side of the Atlantic. Even in the Old

World cholera was not a major pestilence once—not when compared to the pox, bubonic plague, or malaria. In Europe cholera had been known since the fifteenth century, but not in epidemic proportions, such as in its native homes in Asia.

Then, in the early days of the nineteenth century steam displaced sail. In 1807 Robert Fulton's *Clermont* steamed the 150 miles up the Hudson River from New York to Albany in just 32 hours. By 1830 steamships were criss-crossing the seven oceans. The pace of travel by sea quickened. Cholera epidemics appeared in Italy, in France, in the rest of Europe. By 1832, less than a century and a half ago, cholera landed in Quebec.

Travel was slow in the colonies in those days. The cholera stayed in Quebec for a while. By and by it struck up an acquaintaince with French voyageurs, who carried it with them on their canoes and flat-bottomed trading boats up the wide St. Lawrence River and onwards to the Great Lakes. Colonists gave it a ride next on board prairie schooners, the Red River carts of the

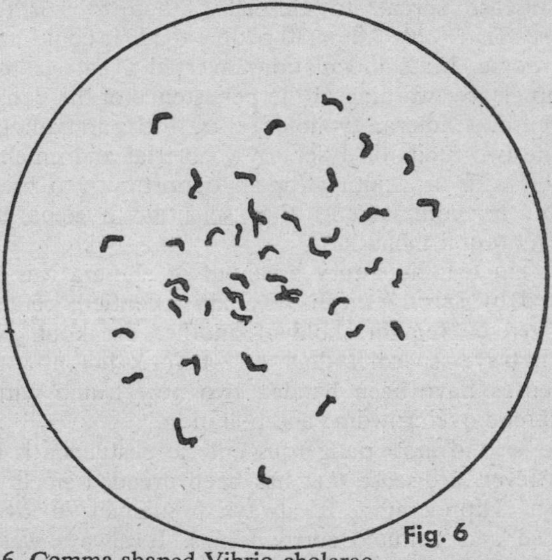

Fig. 6

Fig. 6. Comma-shaped Vibrio cholerae.

day, the wagon trains. The U.S. Cavalry on patrol by the banks of the mighty Mississippi made many an unscheduled bivouac because of it. Smart Yankee traders were not immune. They carried it south. In 1840 cholera struck New York City, where 4,500 people died.

Today one is tempted to think that cholera and the other enteric pestilences should be ghosts of the past. All these varieties of enteritis are thoroughly understood. All are spread by infection of water supplies. Since all water destined for consumption is purified by municipalities under the supervision of Public Health authorities, there should theoretically no longer be any epidemics. Vaccines are available. There should not even be individual cases, not even in such endemic localities as Naples, Italy, about which beautiful city there was a saying current for two centuries: "See Naples and die!"

The 1973 cholera epidemic that originated once again in Naples has effectively displaced all complacency. In that year there were some 500 cases in Italy. The disease spread to Germany, then to northern Europe. True, only 20 or 30 people died. It could have been worse. Mass inoculations averted a catastrophe. But no clearer warning of the persistence of the danger is needed. Cholera, typhoid fever, the paratyphoids, and the two kinds of dysentery (bacterial and amebic) are still with us, waiting for an opportunity to break out of the confinements that scientific hygiene has thrown around them.

The nineteenth-century breakout of cholera was facilitated by speedy travel. The late twentieth century may well be the threshold of another breakout. Not only is travel speedier than ever before, but now the pestilences have been handed two new trump cards: widespread overcrowding and pollution.

The second most dangerous enteric pestilence is typhoid fever, a disease that has been dreaded since the days of Hippocrates. It always flourished in overcrowded and polluted surroundings. It always was a camp follower of war. In each year of the American

Civil War 1,000 participants out of 100,000 died from it; and this was not unexpected. Then came the recognition of its cause. By the time of World War I, the death incidence dropped to 5 in 100,000.

All enteric pestilences are similar. Except for amebic dysentery each is caused by a similarly behaving kind of entamoeba, all these diseases are contracted by drinking water or by eating uncooked fruit or vegetables or shellfish contaminated with water in which there are live bacteria. All these bacteria are easily killed by efficient treatment of sewage; in other words, the diseases are contracted by drinking or eating raw sewage.

In cholera the most profound symptom is profuse, thin, watery diarrhea. The stools are flecked with fragments of necrotic bowel lining and look like rice water. Severe dehydration and electrolyte disturbances (see Section 8) soon appear.

In bacterial dysentery the main symptom is also diarrhea. The stools are numerous and odorless and consist almost entirely of blood and mucus (red currant jelly stools).

Amebic dysentery is more chronic—slow in onset and prolonged. The stools are large, offensive, and streaked with blood and mucus (anchovy sauce stools).

In typhoid the intensity of the fever, with malaise, a desire for sleep, headache, and abdominal pain often overshadow bowel symptoms. Rose spots appear on the skin.

In paratyphoid, headache and abdominal pain are the major symptoms. Meningitis is common.

What can you to to protect yourself and your family from enteric pestilence?

First, when traveling in hot climates, be sure to take all necessary inoculations. Some of these are not pleasant, but any such unpleasantness is only a small sample of what the disease itself can do. Make certain that you receive reinoculations at necessary time intervals.

Second, closer to home, do your part in preventing and clearing pollution. The greatest danger in North

America today exists in the expensively motorized, overcrowded shanty towns that go by the name of campgrounds. Insist on there being properly constructed washrooms in all of them, especially in shoestring operated private ones. Resist the temptation to use the bushes when washrooms are occupied. If you do have to relieve yourself in the open, dig a small hole first, then cover your excreta with dirt. Do not chew your fingernails. Wash your hands. Do not empty your recreational vehicle's holding tank into a roadside ditch. Support legislation dealing with the disposal of effluents from pleasure boats. When afloat, do not use the "bucket n' chuck it" sanitation method.

When building a cottage obey scrupulously all ordinances pertaining to the construction of privies and to the building of septic tank disposal fields.

Do not oppose municipal expenditures on sewage disposal plants.

What can you do if there is an outbreak of enteric pestilence in your locality?

First, do not panic. Get yourself inoculated as soon as possible, but even then follow this simple rule: You can stay untouched by the disease, even if you are not inoculated, by not drinking raw water and not eating anything that has been in contact with raw water.

Boil all drinking water. Cook all fruit and vegetables. Avoid shellfish altogether. If cooking the drinking water is not practical, disinfect it with water sterilization tablets (obtainable from any store that sells camping equipment). If you cannot get water sterilization tablets, use ordinary household chlorine-type bleach. Add enough bleach to the water so that it just smells of chlorine. Let it stand for two hours, longer if possible, before use.

What can you do if you happen to be in a locality where an enteric pestilence is prevalent and you yourself develop a bout of diarrhea?

Again, do not panic. Your diarrhea may be due to

any of the other causes described in this book. Follow the instructions detailed in the section on gastroenteritis (Section 19). Follow the instructions on cooking and disinfecting drinking water detailed above. Dispose of your own stools in as sanitary a manner as possible. Wash your hands often. Secure a sample of your stool —an ounce or less in any clean glass jar will do fine— and get in touch with a doctor.

23. Drugs, Chemicals, Poisons

Hundreds of thousands of years ago some unsung genius noted that eating certain plants produced rather unexpected results. One such result might have been purgation. The primitive genius put two and two together, and remembered. The next time he himself or perhaps someone else in his tribe suffered from constipation, he searched the forest for the same plant, gathered its leaves, and initiated the very first therapeutic trial of a "new" drug. In the process he founded the art of medicine, originated the science of pharmacology, and laid down the basis of the drugged society.

Today billions of drug users consume thousands of tons of various drugs daily. The benefits of licit drug use are enormous. The dangers of even legitimate drug use are formidable.

Drugs can harm you in many ways. As far as their effect on your intestinal tract is concerned, they can give rise to very acute, or else to debilitating, low-grade but prolonged gastroenteritis, with vomiting and diarrhea, through any of the following mechanisms:

1. Toxicity. A drug acts as a drug only if it is taken in suitable doses. Generally adult doses are larger than doses for children, but in the case of some drugs the reverse is true. Also, the dose suitable in the presence of one disease is not suitable in another disease, or even in different stages of the same disease.

Additionally, each drug has a local action on the stomach and the intestine, as well as a general action on the whole of the body. Arsenic, the darling drug of Victorian society, in small doses has a stimulating action on the stomach—it aids digestion. In larger doses it acts as a severe protoplasmic poison and produces copious and repeated watery diarrhea just like the pestilence cholera. Its general action includes itching of the eyelids, bronchitis, skin rashes, and muscular paralysis. Arsenic is no longer used as a drug but is present in many bug killers and garden sprays. The poison labels on these products mean what they say.

2. Cumulative toxicity. This effect occurs when a repeatedly taken drug is not completely eliminated from the body by the time each successive dose is taken. A buildup of drug concentration takes place in body tissues. A good example is furnished by the heart drug digitalis. When its use is prolonged, its effects may gradually become poisonous, involving not only the heart but also the intestinal tract, with nausea, diarrhea, and vomiting.

3. Idiosyncrasy. People react to the same doses of the same drugs in different ways. An individual may show an excessive reaction to a normal dose (hypersusceptibility)—for example, many small children are unduly susceptible to the action of opium compounds: or a diminished reaction (tolerance) for example, there are people who can tolerate more booze than others. The term "idiosyncrasy" also applies in the case of a person who develops a totally unexpected reaction to a drug—for example, a stomach hemorrhage from aspirin.

4. *Intolerance.* Some people cannot tolerate even the smallest dose of some drugs. Meperidine (Demerol, Winthrop) is a potent narcotic used for the relief of severe pain. There are people in whom it produces vomiting.

5. *Side effects.* Many drugs produce unwanted and undesired effects in addition to the desired effects. This happens very often indeed. Phenylbutazone (Butazolidin, Geigy) and Indomethacin (Indocid, MSD) are topnotch drugs for the relief of the pain of arthritis and rheumatism. Unfortunately, they are apt to irritate the intestine, with the production of a drug-induced, chemical gastroenteritis. They occasionally have other side effects, on the blood.

6. *Allergy.* True allergy is an altered reaction of some body tissues when excited by allergens or antigens. In popular parlance the term has come to mean any unusual reaction to drugs, chemicals of all sorts, molds, plants, fungi. True allergy is never something you are born with but is always acquired as a result of the use of or exposure to certain substances. You can live half your life without being allergic to penicillin, for instance. Then one day you get a skin rash or diarrhea or asthma from it, and henceforth every time you are exposed to penicillin, the reaction is liable to recur and to be worse. Penicillin can give rise to diarrhea by a different mechanism too (see Section 26).

7. *Withdrawal.* These problems are the price some people pay for becoming habituated to certain drugs. The worst mental and intestinal withdrawal symptoms occur in narcotic addicts. Less severe but still prolonged and unpleasant looseness of the stools is experienced by people who have become habituated to the use of headache remedies containing codeine. When deprived of it, they experience many loose stools daily for weeks, even months.

Drug induced gastroenteritis is a very common disease indeed. If you suddenly or gradually develop the symptoms described in the introduction to the section on gastroenteritis (Section 19), if you are presently taking a drug—any drug or any combination of drugs—and if your illness pattern does not quite fit the descriptions of other causes of diarrhea and vomiting detailed in other sections, then chances are that the drugs which you are taking are causing it.

The cornerstone of treatment is to stop taking the offending drug. If this is a prescription item, then check with your doctor first. If it is something you bought over the counter, then quit using it cold turkey. If your gastroenteritis is at all severe, then additionally follow the instructions on treatment in Section 19.

24. Booze

Some pleasant evening while pulling the tab off a can of beer, raise it in a toast to the men of Sennar, of the land which the Bible calls Babylon, and which today is called Iran. Close your eyes, switch your imagination into Technicolor, and picture them saying to one another: "Come, let us bake bricks to make stone and let us use bitumen for mortar, and let us build ourselves a city and a tower with its top in the heavens." Take a sip of your beer. Savor its taste. You are drinking the most ancient alcoholic beverage known to man, invented by these same men of the valleys of Babel, some 6,000 years ago. While you are doing this, also reflect upon the coincidence that their particular building project came to nothing.

The effects of alcohol on the mind are well known. Also important are its effects on the intestine.

Alcohol is one of the very few substances which are absorbed into the bloodstream unchanged from any point in the intestinal tract. In practice this means absorption from the mouth, from the throat, from the stomach, and from the small intestine. Locally small, well-diluted doses of alcohol have a stimulating effect. They increase the intestinal blood circulation, help in the passage of intestinal gas, aid digestion. In larger, more concentrated doses alcohol irritates with the production of typical pharyngitis, gastritis, and gastroenteritis. A severe alcoholic gastritis can end in a frank and dangerous hemorrhage.

After absorption from the intestine alcohol circulates in the bloodstream. The circulation carries it everywhere, including the brain. Depending on the dose and on your particular reaction to it, this results in your feeling loving or happy or tipsy or fighting mad or depressed. After a while, if you have quit drinking for a time, those feelings pass. What has happened?

What has happened is that your liver has filtered the alcohol out of your blood. It has changed it chemically. In the process it has detoxified its inebriating (toxic) qualities and has extracted and stored its caloric energy for food.

The liver is the filter of your circulation and the food warehouse of your body. Unlike the oil filter in your car, it does not have to be replaced every 6,000 miles. It possesses fantastic self-cleansing properties. If, however, it has to deal with toxins continuously—if you keep drinking day after day, month after month—it too clogs in a process called cirrhosis. It then no longer filters the blood; since the circulation of the blood to the liver is a one-way passage, the stream of blood leading to it backs up. Veins on the periphery of the liver circulation swell, become varicose, eventually burst. The result is another type of gastrointestinal hemorrhage, much more serious than that from an acute alcoholic gastroenteritis. With this type of hemorrhage, with the liver in a state of failure, patients do not usually live long.

When you drink, you do not often drink alcohol as such—your booze is hard liquor, beer, or wine. With hard liquor the effects of the concentrated alcohol predominate. With beer and wine you take in a lot of fluids—mostly water—and vegetable extracts and chemically complex flavorings. When beer and wine are taken in moderation, the effects of the water and of the vegetable carminatives (see Section 71) balance the effects of the alcohol. Beer and wine in moderation stimulate the intestinal tract, increase the blood circulation to the stomach and intestines, prevent and treat accumulations of gas (see Section 72), and improve digestion. The stools are loosened somewhat. Unless you overindulge, diarrhea does not occur. Beer and wine are consequently important aides in the treatment of constipation, especially in the elderly (see Section 51). People who overindulge commonly do so in two patterns. The man (or woman) who goes on benders insults his stomach to the point where the large amounts of concentrated liquor taken act as a potent irritant and protoplasmic poison. Result is a gross swelling of the mucous lining of the stomach and perhaps a hemorrhage. It is the chronic drinker who gets cirrhosis.

25. Travelers' Diarrhea

The traveler sits and eats nowadays. Hawaii, Mexico, Costa Brava—the sitting begins with a wait in the airport lounge. Paris, Moscow, Hong Kong—it continues in the reclining seat aboard the airplane. Calgary, Tampa, Toronto—travel by car is not different.

Aboard the airplane the dragging hours do not register on the face of any clock. Your own watch is always wrong. Your flight captain obligingly tells you every so many mealtimes to advance its hands so many revolutions, back so many revolutions. Didn't you just eat breakfast? The stewardess is passing out dinner menus. Your stomach is full. It badly needs to move its contents along to make room for the next load of cuisine, which your eyes cannot refuse because your wallet has paid for it already. Your stomach cannot do that very well, unless your colon shifts its contents first.

But your colon balks. It has its own timetable to observe. That timetable is initially slowed by your immobility (see Section 46). Your colon's first reaction is constipation. Eventually, under the press of more eating, your colon is overwhelmed. By then all of you, including your digestive apparatus is tired, exhausted, but finally you safely arrive at your destination. Chances are that by now you are active again, and what is more, you are eating foods to which you are not accustomed. And bingo . . . diarrhea!

Travel upsets your eat-work-recreation-sleep routine, on which regularity depends. Tiredness, overeating, lack of exercise, unusual food and drink, different minerals in the water—all take their toll. The price you pay is initial constipation, followed by diarrhea.

There is another factor. Every living organism develops a resistance to strains of bacteria to which it has been exposed in the past. In other words, you get used to your homegrown germs, much in the same way as the native of Mexico or Germany or China gets used to his. Travel exposes you to a different germ environment, one against which you do not have a defense. These germs then proceed to have a ball, while you suffer. Involved are strains of staph of the food poisoning producing type (see Section 21), strains of colon bacilli (Section 2), various pestilential bacteria (Section 22), and certain molds and fungi. If you unluckily make contact with any of these, your initial constipation-diarrhea episode will then progress along the lines of one of the varieties of gastroenteritis described in the preceding sections.

What can you do about it? You cannot avoid the time zone upsets or the loss of sleep. Sleeping pills are no solution. Drugs are of limited value.

En route you can refuse the extra portions of food, as well as the booze. You can take some hometown baked bread along, even some wife-made sandwiches. Travel with a lunchbox is not romantic; whether you do so should depend on your plans on arrival. If your strategy is to laze in the sun, then take your chances. If you expect to have to take part in important business soon after arrival, then consider the odds. Napoleon might still have lost the battle of Waterloo, even if he had not suffered from diarrhea at the time; as it was, commanding a mounted army while unable to sit on horseback was certainly no asset to him.

If you must eat on the way, then eat sparingly. Do not overload your stomach. If your digestion is otherwise sound, if you are not prone to *any* type of intestinal upsets, then highly seasoned food will do you no harm but may even help (see Section 71). If you must drink on the way, then stick to beer or high-quality wines with your meals, and drink only liqueurs after meals (see Section 71). Do not drink on an empty stomach or before or between meals.

On arrival first get some exercise—walk around the block a few times—then get some rest, if possible. Switch to local foods gradually. Now is the time to avoid highly seasoned foods. Hotels and restaurants everywhere feature an "international bland" cuisine as well as their own exotic specialties. They may not display it prominently on the menu; you may have to ask. Do not drink anything alcoholic at all for a day or two. Avoid also drinking raw (unboiled) water, unpasteurized milk, all hot and fresh breads, all fresh fruit, all tasty tender vegetables, and all fish and shellfish.

After the first two or three days abroad, if the country you are visiting enjoys a high standard of sanitation, you can relax your dietary restrictions almost completely. Avoid eating sweets sold in an obviously unhygienic manner. Wash fresh fruit and produce in copious amounts of water; if there is any garden dirt on them, wash it off with soap; rinse the soap off well. Bring unpasteurized milk to a boil. Eat all meat and fish only well done (to kill tapeworm eggs). Be careful where you swim and keep your mouth shut while swimming.

If you are visiting in hot, tropical, or underdeveloped countries make certain that you are adequately inoculated against all pestilential diseases that prevail there. Avoid wading in swamps and do not swim in unchlorinated water.

If you are an important politician or a top business executive and you know that you will not be able to rest before you are scheduled to take part in official functions, then take along a complete supply of accustomed foods, as well as your private cook. This goes also for people who travel by private or company airplanes. Your diplomatic hosts as well as the big hotels expect this from you and will be prepared to accommodate.

There is just one drug that is of use in the prevention

of travelers' diarrhea (gastroenteritis type). It bears the forbidding chemical name of iodochlorhydroxyquin, but is better known under its Ciba trade name of Vioform in the United States. It is a good specific remedy against the disease amebic dysentery, and in addition it is also effective against a wide spectrum of other diarrhea-producing germs, including those that produce bacterial dysentery, several varieties of colon bacteria, several kinds of molds, and some fungi. For maximum protection it must be taken for two days before the expected time of exposure to the infection. The adult dose is two tablets daily. Like all drugs, it also has its disadvantages. It must not be continued for more than four weeks. Since it contains iodine, it is not suitable for anyone who suffers or has ever suffered from any disease of the thyroid gland or goiter or anyone who is allergic to iodine. Pregnant women should not take it either. Allergies to it, especially skin rashes, do occur.

Notwithstanding the above reservations, iodochlorhydroxyquin is a good drug. It cannot and will not take the place of the common-sense precautions against contacting infectious gastroenteritis outlined previously, but when taken as an additional protection, especially when traveling in hot climates, it can make the difference between enjoyment and misery.

Treatment

Travelers' diarrhea consists of three phases. First, there is a phase of constipation brought on by immobility, aided by overeating and tiredness. Second, there comes the reaction and revolt of the overloaded gut: the actual diarrhea bout. Third, in some cases only, there may come a bout of infectious gastroenteritis from ingesting germs to which you have not been exposed before and against which you have not previously acquired a resistance.

In actual experience a traveler may suffer through all

three phases, but he may be troubled just by one or another.

If your initial constipation phase proves unduly troublesome and persistent and especially if you are prone to be "costive" at the best of times, then this alone may need treatment. Read the sections of this book that deal with constipation. As far as specific remedies are concerned, read the section on immobility constipation (Section 46) and the section on salt laxatives (Section 56).

In the treatment of the second phase—the phase of reactive diarrhea—the best thing to do initially is to get on with it. Your overloaded colon deserves the chance to empty itself, even to have one or two temper tantrums in protest against the insults and injustices you have inflicted upon it. If the diarrhea lasts too long, and if you can get a doctor's prescription, then take next a bowel sedative such as Elixir Donnatal (made by Robins) or a dose of paregoric (camphorated tincture of opium). These two work the best. If you cannot get a doctor's prescription, take full doses of one of the kaolin and pectin preparations listed in Section 19. If these or similar mixtures are not available to you, then eat nothing, drink only boiled water or weak tea with a little sugar added, and follow the other steps described for the treatment of gastroenteritis (Section 19).

If the timing and the persistence of your diarrhea suggest that it is in the nature of a germ-produced gastroenteritis, then read the sections on this subject (Sections 19-21) and follow the treatments given there.

26. Antibiotic Diarrhea

A thousand years ago, in the then-brand-new East European country of Poland, a novel and effective method of wound treatment came into use. It consisted of packing wounds with a mixture of bread molds and cobwebs. Ten centuries later the germ-killing powers of a green mold called *Penicillium notatum* were discovered by England's Sir Alexander Fleming.

Today some thirty different kinds of antibiotics are in common use. All are derived from molds and fungi. Some, like penicillin, are bacteriocidal—that is, they have the power to kill bacteria. Others, like the tetracyclines, are bacteriostatic: they can stop bacteria from multiplying, thus giving the body a chance to fight them. Some, such as ampicillin, have a broad spectrum of activity: they kill, or interfere with the reproduction of, many kinds of germs. Others are selective: they are active against only a few. None is completely without disadvantages or dangers. Some, like kanamycin, are very toxic but still very valuable because no other, safer antibiotics exist to take their place.

Antibiotics, especially those with a wide spectrum of activity, produce diarrhea in this manner: They clean up all germs in the intestinal tract within reach, including those that should be there (see Section 2). Once the rightful tenants have thus been evicted, others that normally do not belong there and are not susceptible to the action of the antibiotic make their appearance. The result is an enteritis causing a diarrhea, from what is called an overgrowth of nonantibiotic-susceptible organisms.

The course of such an illness is quite typical. Let us say that you are taking an antibiotic for treatment of a sore throat, cough, or ear infection. On the third or fourth day of antibiotic medication you may or may not be feeling better. But now you also develop abdominal cramps, nausea, and diarrhea. The diarrhea may be low grade but may become worse than the illness for which you took the antibiotic in the first place.

The obvious treatment is to stop taking the antibiotic that is responsible. If your original ailment was slight or is improving, then you are better off to sweat it out and not take any more antibiotics of any kind until your gut is normal again. If your original illness is still not improving, then you will have to switch to a different antibiotic and take treatment for the diarrhea as well.

If your diarrhea proves severe or persistent, then follow the management routine described in Section 19. In addition, it helps to eat cottage cheese and to drink cultured buttermilk, or else to take capsules (for example, Lactinex, made by Hynson, Westcott, Dunning) that contain the kind of bacteria normally found in dairy products. These are called lactobacilli. They are friendly. They do no harm. They take up the place vacated by the evicted normal colon inhabitants and in this way help to control the undesired germs.

Note: Antibiotic diarrhea is not an allergy. If you have once experienced it, it does not necessarily follow that you will suffer from it again. It is possible, however, to develop an allergy to an antibiotic (see Section 14). Antibiotic diarrhea occurs often. True antibiotic allergy that produces a diarrhea is rare.

27. Ulcerative Colitis

Ulcerative colitis is a serious illness in which the lining of the colon becomes inflamed to the point of bleeding and ulcer formation. It starts in one of three ways.

First, there may be a gradually developing looseness of the bowels, which goes on either continuously or as a series of attacks. Second, there may be a series of bouts from the start, with diarrhea-free intervals. Each bout is blamed on something different—overeating, travel, food poisoning, drinking, and so on. An explosive onset of a diarrhea that immediately is severe and lasting is the third way.

Once established, the prolonged diarrhea either is continuous or comes in successive waves of deterioration and partial improvement. The stools are watery and contain blood and pus. There may be an evacuation every hour of the day and night. The patient may develop fluctuation of the body temperature or else a high fever. He feels weak and tired, loses his appetite, and loses weight. Electrolyte disturbances soon follow (see Section 8). Complications are frequent.

The cause of this disease is completely unknown. Bacterial infections have been blamed for it. Virus infections have been considered. It is not a form of cancer. It may be a form of extreme allergy, but if so, the exciting allergen has not been recognized. It may have a psychogenic cause. It is not a neglected disease. It is the subject of intensive investigations in many medical centers around the world. At the time of writing, at least forty different theories about its cause have been advanced; none has been proved. The day is hopefully coming when the cause will be known, but to date, it is still an enigma.

As far as treatment is concerned the picture is not black, for the vast majority of patients can be helped to regain good health. Effective treatment exists both by medical means (medicines, drugs) and by surgery. But the treatment is complex and a description of it is outside the scope of this book.

28. Crohn's Disease

Crohn's disease is also called regional ileitis or regional colitis. Its cause is just as unknown as is the cause of ulcerative colitis (Section 27). It differs from ulcerative colitis in that it involves one or more distinct regions of the bowel, not the whole of the colon. The region most commonly affected is the last two feet of the small intestine.

Crohn's disease occurs in various forms, only one of which is characterized by diarrhea. It may strike suddenly, like appendicitis. It may block off the bowel like a cancer, but it is not a form of cancer.

Its treatment is usually surgery, with generally good results. It can, however, recur, in which case another operation often offers a fair to good chance of cure.

29. Diarrhea as a Symptom of Other Diseases

A large number of diseases may start with a bout of diarrhea or else the diarrhea is but one of other symptoms. Among the many are some tropical diseases, diseases of the metabolism, and poisoning with many substances (see Section 23). Peptic ulcer disease sometimes produces diarrhea, as does gall bladder inflammation. Hepatitis is a common illness, in which the loose stools are yellow; jaundice follows. In certain kinds of heart disease the blood flow to the intestine is impaired, and constipation or diarrhea results; sometimes the two alternate. A looseness of the bowels can be the first sign of cancer of the intestine, especially if blood is mixed with the stool. Diseases of the thyroid gland cause diarrhea at times, together with nervousness, loss of weight, and the appearance of a lump (goiter) in the neck.

All these diverse illnesses have one thing in common: a change in accustomed bowel habits. As was discussed in Section 5, this is more important than the diarrhea.

30. Overflow Diarrhea

This condition occurs at the extremes of life: in small children and in the very aged. It is characterized not so much by diarrhea occurring in attacks or bouts but by a passive flow of liquid fecal material that leaks out of the anus and soils underwear and bedding. Mothers should watch out for it. It is definitely not caused by the child being too lazy to go to the bathroom. The child cannot help it, and neither can the senior citizen in his wheelchair.

It is, in fact, not diarrhea at all but an extreme form of constipation called fecal impaction. The constipated stool forms into a ball the size of a softball or larger and lies deep in the pelvic part of the colon, only an inch or so up from the anus. It is much too large to pass through the anus. It lies there like a rock. Liquid fecal material trickles and flows around it and in this way finds a route to leak through the anal orifice.

More details about this condition will be found in the section dealing with constipation in the elderly (Section 51).

Treatment must consist of initially breaking up that ball of hard feces and evacuating it, then of regulating the bowel function so that it does not recur. Laxatives are useless and can do grave damage. The evacuation must be done from below, using suitable suppositories and enemas (see Section 59) to soften the hard mass. At times manual breaking up of the rocks, not a pleasant task, is necessary. Using a plastic or rubber glove insert a finger into the rectum and with perseverance divide the huge lump into pieces, then extract the pieces one by one. If you yourself cannot do it, then a doctor or nurse or a trained orderly will have to do it.

Regulation of bowel function to prevent a recurrence is described in the sections on constipation in Part III.

PART III. CONSTIPATION

31. Introduction

A dictionary defines constipation as "the infrequent and difficult passage of hard, dry stools". No one quarrels with the second half of this definition. Hard, dry stools often are difficult to pass. There are, however, many misconceptions about what constitutes an "infrequent" passage.

Most people use the toilet once or twice daily, but there are perfectly healthy individuals who have an evacuation only once every two or three days. This type of infrequency does not necessarily mean constipation. As was described in Section 3, a "good" daily movement empties completely the left (descending) side of the colon (see Fig. 3). This is achieved in one go by some people, in two sessions by others. Since the main function of the colon is the extraction of water, the longer the stool stays in the bowel, the drier and harder it becomes. Consequently folks who have an evacuation only once every two or three days pass relatively smaller amounts than people who do so daily. Their stools are also drier and harder, but as long as the passage is not painful and not difficult, they do not suffer from constipation. If you are one of these people, you can quit reading right here.

Frequently in these cases the stools are also large in diameter. Some modern plumbing fixtures do not allow such bulky stools to be flushed. Toilets become blocked, with rather unpleasant consequences. The "treatment" in these instances is not to resort to laxatives but to replace the toilet.

There are many popular misconceptions about a supposedly poisonous effect of stools that are not passed at least once daily. This is nonsense. If your pattern is to use the toilet every second or third day, if your experience is that this does not result in a difficult passage of stools, if you feel healthy, then fine. Do not get carried away by advertisements that tout some laxative or other that promote, "regularity." You are "regular" already. By definition, you are not even constipated.

Things are different, however, if you do not feel healthy with infrequent bowel movements. An overfull, distended colon generates reflex nerve impulses that are translated in the brain as feelings of bloating or of an enlargement of the whole of the abdomen. You feel uncomfortably big about the waistline. This feeling causes you to gag. You try to belch. The mechanism of belching is remarkable in that to do so voluntarily you must first swallow a mouthful of air to distend your esophagus (the foodpipe from mouth to stomach). Then there must follow a contraction of the walls of your stomach, which must be synchronized with a relaxation of your stomach inlet. All this means that to effect a successful belch of, say, two mouthfuls of air, you must first swallow one mouthful of air. If there is no surplus air in your stomach or if your timing is a bit off, the result will be that you have swallowed air and not belched up any. Do that a few times and your stomach and intestines will really fill up. You will feel, and by then you will be, more bloated than ever.

Constipation can be the first stage, and in another sense the cause, of a blockage or obstruction of the intestine. If unrelieved, it next causes a backing up of intestinal contents. This is experienced as a feeling of nausea. If still not relieved it becomes vomiting. Headache of a peculiar sickly quality soon supervenes, together with backache, and a general feeling of malaise. The tongue, which is the only part of the intestinal tract that is easily inspected, becomes furred with a thick, yellowish brown coating. The breath becomes offensive. The swollen abdomen becomes painful and tender (painful on pressure).

Complete bowel obstruction from constipation, which in such a case would be called a fecal impaction (without overflow—see (Section 30), is uncommon. It occurs most often in very young children and in the very elderly (see Sections 30 and 51).

32. The Work of the Intestine

The twenty-odd feet of the small intestine and the five-odd feet of the large intestine are not just a system of plumbing tubes fixed immovably in one position. They move, flow, writhe, and churn, all the time. Also, the intestines do not just hang from the diaphragm and are not just attached to the anus like a free-form futuristic pole-lamp fixture. All along their entire length they are attached to the backbone area of the abdomen by a soft membrane that carries within it blood vessels, lymph vessels, and nerves.

The intestines themselves are fleshy tubes. Their walls consist of several layers. Innermost is a layer of mucous membrane studded with millions of tiny projections called villi. Each villus is the terminal for one artery, which brings blood to it, and the starting point of one vein, which carries blood away from it to the liver. The villi are covered with cells, which do the actual work of extracting nutrients from the chemical mash into which your steak and your bread and butter have been transformed by the action of the intestinal juices described in Section 2. Surrounding the mucous membrane layer are several coats of muscle tissue. This is a different muscle than the one in your biceps: Its fibers contract and relax in a definite pattern, but unless you are a Yogi, its contractions are not subject to your voluntary control. You cannot hold your intestines still as you can your arm or leg. You cannot make them churn at will, which is unlike your ability to kick a football or to cuddle your spouse.

The intestinal muscles react to stimuli. The most important of these is the presence of a food mash within the intestinal tract, but they also react to the sight, smell, even talk of food. The twitching and growling of a hungry stomach is surely known to everyone. They are also influenced by such emotions as joy, tension, anxiety, and worry. And they are influenced by drugs.

The movements of the intestine produced by the involuntary action of their muscles fall into five patterns. Together they are called peristalsis.

Peristalsis

The most obvious movements of the intestine are called wave peristalsis. They are seen daily by every surgeon who operates in the abdomen. They consist of a succession of waves of contractures preceded by relaxations that milk and propel the food mash onward. The average peristaltic wave travels along the bowel at a speed of one to two inches per minute. When the intestine is irritated, as in food-poisoning diarrhea, the peristaltic waves travel faster. When there is a blockage of the intestine the peristaltic waves become disorganized and may take a reverse direction. In constipation from any cause, the waves are slowed.

The second easily recognized intestinal movements are those of segmentation. These are rhythmical local contractions that for a time divide the intestine into segments.

The third type of peristalsis is churning for the purpose of mixing intestinal contents.

The fourth type of movements are pendulum motions. These can be seen only on x-ray examinations. Their significance is not completely known.

The large intestine (colon) exhibits a fifth type of movements not shown by the small intestine. Called mass movements, they are most marked in the transverse and descending parts of the colon—that is, in those parts of the large intestine that deal with a less liquid mash and with stools. Occurring only two or three times in each twenty-four hours, they consist of a powerful contraction wave, preceded by a relaxation, of up to two feet of colonic length in front of it. They serve to push a whole two-foot length of colonic contents onward to the rectum.

You feel a peristaltic mass movement of your colon first as a sensation of rectal fullness, next as an urge to use the toilet. If a bathroom is handy, you consciously allow the movement to continue and assist it by a maneuver that increases your intra-abdominal pressure in the act known as "bearing down" or "pushing."

If the opportunity is not right, you cannot stop the colonic mass movement but you can suppress the urge to go. This is known as bowel training. It results in your rectum remaining full until such time as using a bathroom is possible. If the urge to defecate is repeatedly suppressed, however, then the conscious awareness of your rectum being full gradually decreases. This mechanism produces one constipation pattern.

Gastrocolic Reflex

As mentioned earlier in this section, intestinal muscles that produce peristaltic movements react to stimuli. One such stimulus that acts on the large bowel is the very important gastrocolic reflex.

It works this way: When food distends the previously empty stomach and also when food leaves the stomach to enter the previously empty first part of the small intestine called the duodenum (see Section 2), it generates a nerve reflex that acts as a stimulus on the colon. The colon responds with a mass movement.

This reflex is influenced by the speed with which the stomach empties itself after eating; since an excess of fat in the food makes for slow stomach emptying, the reflex does not occur, or else is weak, if the meal was greasy. Similarly, the reflex is also absent or weak if stomach emptying is delayed by emotion—love, hate, excitement, tension, worry.

The gastrocolic reflex is effective only a few times during the day. It is strongest after breakfast—that is when the stomach was initially quite empty, when the breakfast meal is bulky yet not greasy, and light, and when the cares of the day have not yet made a big impression on the mind. Using the toilet after breakfast utilizes the gastrocolic reflex to the fullest. Ignoring it and suppressing a call to stool at that time of the day repeated over many years abolishes it and contributes to a second chronic constipation pattern.

33. Faulty Diet Causes Constipation

A few years ago the subject of nutrition was cut and dried. There were no disagreements. Problems such as undernutrition, malnutrition, scurvy, pellagra, and beriberi were reduced to a simple arithmetic of counting calories and weighing vitamins and minerals. Councils of nutrition were set up in the U.S. and many other countries, and established recommended daily allowances of calories, proteins, fats and carbohydrates, as well as various vitamins and minerals. Their findings were published in neat little tables that detailed what every man, woman, and child should eat every day. As a subject of vigorous scientific inquiry the science of nutrition died.

In the last few years it has become apparent that the subject of nutrition is not dead. True, gross malnutrition leading to such diseases as rickets and scurvy can be prevented by following the recommendations of the nutritional councils. But other problems have arisen—problems such as obesity, which is one of the most serious continent-wide health hazards in North America and which stubbornly is not conquered by any counting of calories; cardiovascular disease, which has been increasing in incidence from year to year and now deserves the name of a pandemic, and which may be related to the recommended diet; cancer, which claims ever more lives and may be related to some allowed diet additives; and constipation, which has not received the attention it merits as yet but makes life miserable for millions of people and is certainly related to diet.

The nutritional councils' tables are updated every five years, but they have not, to my knowledge, met again for the purpose of a major reexamination of their recommendations. In the meantime there has been no shortage of both serious and faddist diet innovations. For example, Dr. Atkins' Diet Revolution has been investigated by a Senate select committee but deserves a much wider, impartial study. The controversial teachings of nutritionist Adele Davis have never been evaluated properly. The findings and claims of Drs. E. V. and W. E. Shute about the importance of vitamin E have been largely ignored. The views of Nobel Prize winner Dr. Linus Pauling about the importance of vitamin C in the prevention and treatment of the common cold have been treated as a thorn in the comfortable hide of organized medicine. The organic food diet and megavitamins similarly have not been considered.

This book is about digestion, not about diets, but in the context of the problem of constipation—the number 1 problem of digestive disturbances today—the question of diet is paramount.

The nutritional councils teach that, to be health promoting, the daily diet must comprise certain recommended amounts of protein, fat, minerals, carbohydrate, and vitamins. I do not disagree that these items are needed. I question the amounts recommended. In addition I question the nutritional councils' omission of any mention of roughage in their tables and their underemphasis on the importance of water. I question most their action of laying down set figures: so many grams of protein for men of this age, so many milligrams of vitamin C for women of that age. People are individuals. I have yet to meet two men or two women or two boys or two girls of the same age whose body needs are exactly the same.*

The nutritional councils' tables are of great value, but only for purposes of a baseline for the calculation of data applicable in individual cases.

* The nutritional councils' tables are footnoted to the effect that the dietary allowances are intended to meet the needs of healthy individuals. The term "healthy" is not defined. The World Health Organization defines health as "a state of complete physical, mental and social well being, and not merely the absence of disease and infirmity."

34. Eat Enough Protein

Too much protein in the diet results in bacterial putrefaction of the intestinal contents (see Section 4). The stools in such cases are loose, dark, and foul smelling. Too little protein results in the opposite; the stools are pale, with little smell, hard and dry and difficult to pass, that is, the person is constipated.

Food proteins are expensive; however, for the purposes of nutrition it matters little if the meat you eat is steak or hamburger. Apart from soybeans, the cheapest protein food is fish—in fact, seafood of all sorts is excellent protein for the bowel.

The evidence of the efficacy of a high-protein diet in chronic constipation is overwhelming. It comes both from patients and from observation of animals. Consider meat-eating and plant-eating animals. Seagulls eat seafood exclusively; their droppings are liquid. Songbirds, which feed on insects, also have liquid stools. Birds of prey—hawks, eagles, crows, magpies—all have liquid or semi-liquid stools. On the other hand chickens, pigeons, budgerigars which eat mostly grain have firmer droppings and would get really constipated if they did not actively seek out worms and insects or

* The following foods are rich in protein: meat, fish, fowl, eggs, milk, cheese, soybeans. Foods with a fair protein content include nuts, beans, peas, and some grains.

protein rich seeds, and if they did not drink a lot of water.

Mammals that live on plant foods actively search out high protein grains and seeds, which they consume whole—unlike humans who eat their cereals after they have been finely milled and had their protein-rich germ layer sieved out. Even so, rodents—rats, mice, guinea pigs—have firm droppings. Larger plant-eating animals have special mechanisms or methods for the processing of low protein foods. Ruminanes—cattle, deer, sheep, goats, camels—have very special stomachs both for the processing of the roughage that they consume (more about this in section 35) and to compensate for their often protein-poor diet. They also drink a lot of water. For the really good health that goes along with a good digestion and results in superior meat, ranchers "finish feed" their cattle soybeans and other high-protein diet supplements.

The stools of hogs and dogs closely resemble those of humans. Hogs and dogs prefer protein foods. Hog farmers in Iowa and Ontario do not feed their herds on corn alone. They supplement the corn with sorghum, barley, wheat and rye grains, as well as—tankage—ground up animal bones, tendons, intestines.

In the management of habitual or chronic constipation a balanced high-protein diet is a must. As already noted, seafood is the best supplement from this point of view. There is one important exception. Milk and milk solids (condensed milk, dried milk) are high in protein but definitely constipating. If you suffer from constipation avoid drinking milk other than what you add to tea or coffee. Instead eat extra fish. Milk contains, apart from protein, the important minerals calcium and phosphate and vitamins A and D. All these are also found in fish, especially those usually eaten whole—sardines, herring, canned mackerel, canned salmon. For more details see the section on the treatment of chronic constipation (Section 50).

35. Roughage

Dietary roughage is the food-fiber residue not absorbed from the intestinal tract (see Section 3). Although it is not needed by the rest of the body and comes through unchanged in the stools, it is absolutely necessary for the smooth functioning of the whole intestine. It provides the bulk, the mass, around which peristalsis (see Section 32) gets a grip in the mixing, the churning, and the transporting onward of the intestinal contents. Even the strongest, most violent peristaltic contractions are ineffective if the bowel contents are too liquid. This is exactly what happens in diarrhea. Peristalsis is overactive, yet the pressure inside the intestine remains low. The watery bowel contents are eventually sloshed along, but at the cost of an expenditure of intestinal effort felt as a griping, spasmodic pain.

The roughage in your diet is furnished mostly by vegetables. Chemically this is mostly cellulose, the stuff from which paper is made. In foods cellulose is found in the skins of fruit, in the pulp of fruit, in the husks and skins of legumes and grains, and in the stalks and leaf ribs of leafy vegetables. Meat, meat products, and fish also supply some indigestible components but not nearly as much as do vegetables.

Lack of roughage in white flour, in peeled potatoes, and in other highly processed foods that are the staple diet in North America is the most important single cause of constipation today.

There are two kinds of roughage. The desirable kind is found in young, tender, juicy sprouts and leaves and fruits. This kind is easily dealt with by the teeth, the stomach, and the small intestine, which break it up into separate fibers and particles. (In addition, many young, slightly unripe fruits and vegetables also have a natural laxating effect—see Section 53).

The undesirable roughage is present in tough, overripe, and overmature vegetables, which are tough to cook and tough for the intestine to disperse. The teeth, the stomach, and the intestine cannot break it apart, so it comes through in pieces and in chunks. It is found in the skins of ripe tomatoes, apples, peaches, the skins of ripe and dried beans, peas, corn, stalks of woody asparagus, tough leaves of lettuce, raisins and sultanas, even the "dry" pith of overripe and dried-out oranges and grapefruit. All these items come through the intestine essentially intact. They do not contribute to efficiency of peristalsis or to the softness of the stools. If present in large amounts they can solidify stools like the iron rods that are used to reinforce concrete. Every surgeon who performs sigmoidoscopic examinations has seen them. You can see them yourself if you look at your constipated stools carefully.

Grazing animals have special mechanisms for dealing with this kind of roughage. Cattle and other ruminants swallow their feed first and let it soak in the first part of their compound stomachs for several hours, then regurgitate it and chew it again. Horses have special molar teeth adapted for grinding. These teeth have no nerves and never stop growing. They can do justice to tough roughage. You have neither a ruminant stomach nor ever-growing teeth. If you suffer from constipation, avoid tough roughage or soak it overnight, puree it, or put it through a sieve or through a blender. If it is prepared in this way, your intestines will find it almost as useful as that from naturally tender young plants.

36. Drink Enough Water

Lack of water in the body causes dehydration. Absolute dehydration kills rapidly (see Section 8); chronic low-grade dehydration causes sluggishness of all mental and physical body processes and also causes constipation.

By definition, constipation is a condition in which stools are hard and dry and difficult to pass. The less water there is in the intestine, the worse the constipation. Consequently, the first thing you should do if you suffer from constipation is to drink more. The theoretical average adult who is not constipated, does not work, does not sweat, and does not take any salt in his diet requires a minimum of 1,100 ml. (about 1¼ quart) of drinking water daily. The total resting body water requirement per day is double that, but a fair amount of water is also absorbed from food, both from food moisture and from chemical oxidation. The real normal, working, sweating man or woman who likes a bit of salt with his meals requires more, and the normal but constipated adult requires more still. If you avoid taking too much salt with your meals and if you are not severely ill with a heart or kidney ailment, you cannot take too much water; in fact, the more you drink, the less constipated you will be and the better you will feel.

The water you should drink can be in the form of juices, soups, soda, weak coffee or tea, or even beer within reason. Avoid, however, drinking too much milk; milk is constipating (see Section 34). The water can be cold or warm. This matters little. Many older people do well to drink one or two large glasses of hot water with every meal, in addition to all the other liquids consumed per day. You cannot drink too much water.

37. Watch Vitamins and Minerals

A truly balanced diet should supply all nutrients, including all vitamins and minerals, necessary for health. Unfortunately your diet is often less than truly balanced—whether through the increase of needs in illness, by destruction of vitamins in cooking, by your own preferences or fussiness, or because of cost.

Constipation is a symptom of bodily imbalance, not a disease by itself. Some of the factors that can throw your system out of balance have been mentioned in earlier sections. Lack of diet vitamins and minerals is another.

Vitamins and minerals affect nerve and muscle activity, including that of the intestine, which by relaxation and contraction produces peristalsis (see Section 32). Among the many vitamins needed the important ones are vitamin C (ascorbic acid), vitamin B_1 (thiamine), and vitamin B_3 (niacin, nicotinic acid). Of the minerals, the most important is potassium.

Eating a sufficient amount of truly fresh fruit and vegetables should supply your body with plenty of vitamins B and C. Cooking destroys vitamins. Therefore, if most of the fruit you eat has been cooked or canned or if your body needs are increased—for example if you are suffering from an acute or chronic illness—additional vitamins B and C should be taken. Growing children and senior citizens also need supplementary vitamins B and C.

Good, high-potency vitamin supplements are said to be the following:

Albee with C (Robins)
Becotin T (Lilly)
Beforte (Frosst)
Beminal with C Fortis (Ayerst)
B-Totum 500 (Desbergers)
Protobex (Pentagone)
Redoxon-B (Roche)
Stresscaps (Lederle)
Surbex 500 (Abbott)
Unibex-650 (Therapex)

Potassium deficiency is extremely common these days because many people take blood-pressure-lowering drugs, which have the side effect of increasing the loss of potassium in the urine. If you are now taking any high-blood-pressure remedy, you should also compensate for the loss of potassium. The best foods for this are citrus fruit (which are also excellent sources of roughage and of vitamin C), bananas, many meats and fish, peanuts, and almonds.

If you are constipated and feel weak and tired while taking a blood pressure remedy, and if you cannot or will not eat high-potassium foods every day, then ask your doctor about a potassium supplement. Do not take potassium supplements on your own. Potassium in some forms and with some people produces such side effects such as severe stomach and intestinal irritation—in effect, a chemical gastroenteritis (see Sections 19 and 23). Eating high potassium foods is better.

38. Constipation in the Infant and Baby

Throughout this book some conditions are described as common, others as uncommon, still others as rare.

Chances are, if you or your child suffers from something, it is one of the common illnesses. A book such as this, however, must also cover more rare ailments, of which there are many. They are described for the benefit of people who suffer from them or think that they suffer from them. If you or someone in your family experiences symptoms of ill health, do not unduly worry about the rare and terrible things described on these pages. See first, and second, and third, if the symptoms fit one of the common illnesses.

The commonest cause of constipation in the newborn and in the small baby is a formula that is too concentrated (contains too little water) or contains too little sugar or the wrong kind of sugar. In such a case constipation may alternate with diarrhea, which may get worse if you change the formula too frequently. (Read Section 13, on the treatment of diarrhea in the small baby.)

Before changing the formula, experiment by adding a little more water to the mix. For a small baby, the formula is both food and drink. In hot weather or in an overheated home in the winter, the baby needs more water. Between feeds it is often a good idea to offer the baby a few ounces of boiled, cooled water with a little sugar added.

If the baby is still constipated, change the kind of sugar you are using. Generally the darker the sugar (or syrup or molasses), the more laxating it is. So if you have been using ordinary granulated sugar, change first to dark sugar, then, if necessary, to brown sugar. If you have been using syrup, change from a golden one to a dark brown one.

In the unusual case of acute constipation, use a glycerine suppository. Lift the baby's legs and gently insert the suppository into the rectum. Glycerine suppositories are shaped like pencil stubs. Glycerine is a stool softener and a lubricant. It is only minimally irritating, so you can use it repeatedly—within reason—when required. For psychologic reasons do not use the suppository treatment too often in the older child.

Painful movements result from a fissure, or small crack, in the anal verge that becomes infected and is in reality a tiny, linear ulcer. A baby who suffers from it will hold his or her movements back. The treatment for this is described in Section 43.

Infantile colic is dealt with in Section 41.

39. Meconium Ileus

Meconium is a dark, viscid substance that is present in the intestinal tract of the baby at birth (see Section 3). Ileus is a condition in which there is no peristalsis (see Section 32). Meconium ileus is a rare illness of the newborn child in which the bowels do not move.

The problem in this case is that the meconium is so

thick and cohesive that the intestine cannot expel it. As in most diseases, there are less severe and more severe cases. In the less severe case, a series of rectal wash-outs will evacuate it. The more severe case may be helped by an operation in which a surgeon opens into, or injects mucus-dissolving chemicals into loops of the bowel.

Successful treatment of meconium ileus unfortunately is often not the end of the problem. In many instances meconium ileus is but the first manifestation of a generalized abnormality that involves the sweat glands, the mucus-secreting glands of the respiratory tract, of the pancreas, and of other organs of digestion. It is, in other words, often the first sign of celiac disease, described in Section 16.

40. Congenital Megacolon—Hirschsprung Disease

The name "congenital megacolon" means that this condition, in which the newborn baby's colon (large intestine) is oversized, is present from birth. In some families there are more cases of it than are prevalent in the general population, but it is not, strictly speaking, a hereditary disease.

There must clearly be a cause for this condition. In the case of thalidomide babies who were born without arms and without legs, the cause was traced to the drug thalidomide, developed in Germany in the year 1957, and which was then widely advertised and pushed by dozens of drug companies in many countries as a perfectly "safe" sedative. Some time after its introduction one man, Dr. Wiedekind Lenz, observed that there suddenly were more deformed babies being born, and that the deformed births occurred in those areas of Germany in which thalidomide was widely used. What happened next makes an infamous chapter for at least 36 major, so called "ethical" drug combines that pushed the drug, one which the drug manufacturers would dearly love to forget. Dr. Lenz was heaped with abuse and scorn. His professional reputation was besmirched. He was hauled into court. But he was right! For the first time in the history of medicine he proved that a chemical substance, a simple conglomeration of atoms and molecules, influenced the intrauterine development of a human being. He proved his point, and in doing so, opened a new era of research into the causes of other congenital malformations. Now it should be only a matter of time until the causes of other inborn disasters are also recognized.

To date, unfortunately, the cause of congenital megacolon is not yet known. However, there is no mystery about the nature of the defect. It consists of an absence of nerve endings in a segment of the rectum. These nerve endings normally sense if the rectum is full, then trigger the nerve mechanism that produces evacuation. In their absence the brain gets no input and does not know when the bowel is filled. So the colon fills up more and more and stretches until the tummy is huge.

Most cases are not severe. There is constipation. The stools lie in the colon a longer time than is normal, become dry from continuing absorption of moisture (see Section 31), and become hard, pelletlike, and difficult to pass. The stool pellets may fuse into a hard mass, which then either may block the intestinal passage completely or else may allow liquid stools to trickle around it (see the section on constipation with overflow, Section 30).

Luckily, there is treatment available. In severe cases a surgeon can cut out the segment of the bowel that does not contain nerve endings, then rejoin the bowel. This is a delicate and dangerous operation for a six-pound infant to withstand, but it works. In less severe cases it is a question of patient caring nursing and mothering of the infant with the use of suppositories, rectal irrigations, and enemas until the child is old enough to look after his bowels himself. A laxating diet is important from birth (see Section 53). Laxatives help little and may be dangerous. Never give a laxative to your baby unless you have been advised to do so by your doctor.

Things usually improve as the childs gets older. The teenager and the adult who has this problem in some degree should not only read the sections in this book on diet and all other treatments of constipation but should become experts. The problem is real but can be controlled. It need not interfere with anything in life. It need not be a lifelong affliction.

41. The Collicky Baby

A bout of colic starts suddenly. The poor little thing yells, then whimpers miserably, then screams. He or she draws up the legs against the tummy, then stiffens the whole body. The tummy becomes tense, sometimes bloated. The gas is passed by the rectum, but that does not seem to give relief. His pain is obviously intense. Eventually the diapers are filled. The stools are usually constipated and resemble hard little balls but at times are soft and may even be curdy and greenish.

The bout of colic may be short, lasting a few minutes only, or may go on for hours. Nothing seems to help. If the mother picks him up and walks the floor with him, he is quiet for only a minute or so, then the crying, the twisting and turning, the screaming recur. The mother puts the baby back into the crib. The crying continues. The longer it lasts, the greater the chance of vomiting. The vomiting is not, however, prolonged or severe but rather is in the nature of spitting.

The bout of colic may finally pass just as suddenly as it started; baby goes to sleep. Or the bout may subside gradually and be replaced by restlessness, whimpering, and fretting.

The cause of infantile colic is not at all clear. Of the many theories, the most likely postulates that peristalsis has not yet become synchronized by the time of birth so that the contractions of the intestinal muscles do not propel the intestinal contents along smoothly but work against each other. Insufficient burping is a factor. All babies need burping at least once during and more after each feeding. If your baby is prone to suffer from colic, burp him several times during each feeding—every few minutes, if necessary. Also, pay particular attention to see that the feeding nipple is just right, that the baby swallows the absolute minimum of air during feeds. Try using one of the new, polyethylene plastic, collapsible feeding bottles, which do not need to fill with air as the baby sucks the formula. They are excellent in preventing air swallowing. Give the baby small feeds frequently rather than large feeds infrequently. If that still does not help, then switch to a different formula—preferably one based on soybeans and vegetable oils rather than on cows' milk.

Drugs help little. Most of the various commercial gripe-water concoctions available are useless. Avoid giving the baby any laxatives, however persuasive the advertising. If stools are routinely hard, give baby extra water to drink and an extra half-teaspoon to one teaspoon of brown sugar in the formula. If that is still not enough to make the stools soft, offer a teaspoon of prune juice once a day.

A gentle sedative is often the best remedy, both for the baby and for the rest of the family. See your doctor about this.

The condition is distressing but it is not serious. It is self-limiting—that is, it clears spontaneously, whatever the treatment or nontreatment has been, by the age of three or four months.

42. Bowel Training

To understand adult constipation, consider first how children are toilet-trained. From generation to generation, the method has not changed. You were trained like this; if you now have children, this is how you train them. There are four main steps.

1. Catch as catch can
2. Regularity
3. Opportunity
4. Visceral learning

"Catch as catch can" is the name of the game played by mothers and one- or two-year-old toddlers. The child gives a signal—a faraway look, an expression of intense concentration, a sudden quietness, a pause in play. Mother soon learns what this means and comes running with the potty. She misses the event sometimes but gradually is more and more successful. If all goes according to schedule, sooner or later the child gives the signal in time. Accidents still happen, but less frequently. Then a whole physiological and psychological chain reaction sets in. Mother expresses her pleasure when the BM is caught. The child reacts to that expression of pleasure and tries to duplicate it on a subsequent occasion. He slowly gives up the babyish psychological idea that the bowel movement is his own property and begins not to mind its being taken away. By and by the child begins to like being clean, begins to like wearing pants instead of diapers.

At about this time bowel training shifts emphasis from catch as catch can to regularity. Mother sits the toddler on the potty at regular intervals, hopefully preferably after a meal, so as to take advantage of the gastrocolic reflex, described in Section 32. Success follows.

The next stage of training consists of learning to take advantage of a suitable opportunity. This now becomes a do-it-yourself project on the part of the child. Mother still helps, of course, by serving as the child's memory. This stage comes much later than catch as catch can or regularity, usually at the preschool or grade school entrance age, sometimes later. The child learns that certain times and certain occasions are just not convenient for having bowel movements. Putting up a finger in class may be frowned upon by the teacher. Other boys and girls may make fun of the child who has to leave class or has to quit playing. The child who has learned his regularity lesson well and who has become accustomed to using the toilet at home during nonschool hours is obviously well ahead here.

Visceral learning takes place all along, during the training process. The concept is new. It implies that the thinking, conscious human mind has an influence on the so-called involuntary nervous system—that is, on the parts of your brain that control peristalsis, heartbeat, blood pressure, body temperature, body balance, and so on. Visceral learning influences the timing of twice- or thrice daily colonic mass movements and the timing of gastrocolic reflexes (see Section 32), so that they occur only at times convenient for you. With its help you can sit for hours, if need be, while working, playing bridge, or attending a big formal dinner, which would otherwise surely excite your gastrocolic reflex, with neither gas nor a "call" to the bathroom spoiling the affair for you.

It seems that visceral learning is something that can be consciously developed far beyond anything that you pick up as you just simply live. It can be used to control hunger painlessly and in this way used to control weight. According to psychologist Dr. Neal Miller, it can be used to control one's blood pressure—without pills. According to Menninger Foundation's Dr. Elmer Green, it is of use in treating migraine. It seems certain that we have not heard everything about it yet, that it may become a key to the treatment of many bowel problems.

43. Obstacles to Bowel Training

There is more to bowel training than just the end of messy diapering. As Dr. Benjamin Spock points out, for the infant it marks a giant step in development, the step from babyhood to childhood. Psychologically, for the first time in life, your child attempts and succeeds at a complicated task. Success stamps his or her subconscious with the memory of achievement through persistence, of an obligation accepted and carried out. Incomplete success, on the other hand, especially if impressed on the memory by scoldings and expressions of disgust, can be the start of a pattern of repeated failures in later life, can sow the seeds of insecurity and a belief that nothing that he or she attempts will ever turn out quite right.

Two of these are organic and three are psychological.

The first common obstacle to bowel training is an unsuitable diet. A constipating diet is bad enough; a diet that produces bouts of gastroenteritis or causes alternating diarrhea and constipation is worse.

The second common cause of training problems is illness. Major illness causes major setbacks. Minor illness, even a cold, also has an effect. Frequent bowel ailments are diaper rashes, fissures, and worms.

Diaper rashes should be prevented rather than treated. You cannot change the diapers too often. Boil the washed diapers to get rid of ammonia. Wash the baby's buttocks with lots of soap and water. Use a lanolin-containing skin cream. For an established diaper rash, the best treatment is to let the baby sleep on his tummy, with the irritated behind exposed to the air.

If the baby holds his stool back until it becomes hard, then passes it crying with pain and perhaps also with a little blood, the cause is usually a fissure. Gently pull the buttocks apart. You will see the fissure, or perhaps several fissures, as tiny, reddened splits of the anal verge. Fissures start as the result of a passage of a hard, bulky stool. The splits become infected. At every subsequent bowel movement the tiny tears are pulled apart again.

Treat fissures by extrastrict cleanliness. Wash right inside the anal dimple. Carefully rinse off all soap. Adjust the diet with extra brown sugar or extra juices so that the stools are quite soft but without producing diarrhea. If that does not work, use a glycerine suppository daily or even twice daily. Do not use laxatives. If the use of suppositories is not effective, see your doctor about advice on how to stretch the anus and about special suppositories or creams.

Worms appear when the child plays in the dirt—as

all kids do—then puts the dirty fingers in his mouth. Worms are not "nice" but are not a tragedy. The commonest are pinworms, also called threadworms. They crawl outside the anus at night to deposit their eggs and cause itching and scratching. You can easily tell if your child suffers from them. Take a pencil, wrap around it some adhesive tape, such as Scotch tape, with the sticky side outside. When the child is asleep, gently press and wipe the side of the pencil with the adhesive tape on it between the child's buttocks. Take the pencil to a good light. You will see, stuck to the adhesive, bits of fluff from diapers or pajama pants. Among the cotton threads you will see some, about one-fourth inch long, that slowly wave and move.

Roundworms look much like earthworms. They are up to nine inches long and appear in the stools. Unless there are very many of them, they cause surprisingly little trouble.

You can buy worm remedies without a prescription in some areas. They work well. Some of the older, prescription worm remedies are toxic. Do not exceed the dose stated on the label.

Of the three common psychological obstacles to bowel training, the most important is too much parental pressure. Some children are ready for training as soon as they can sit up on the potty unsupported. For most of them the right age to start is between nine and twelve months. Bowel training takes time. It is rarely finished before the child's second birthday and may take much longer. Relapses, called balking, are common. The important thing is not to force the child. If the baby balks, quit sitting him on the potty for a few weeks, then start again.

The second common psychological obstacle to bowel training is too little parental pressure. This occurs when parents take the advice not to force their children too literally. The parent must be a benevolent dictator at times. This question is fully dealt with by Dr. Benjamin Spock in his book *Baby and Child Care*.

The third common psychological obstacle to bowel

training is "nerves." The baby's intestinal tract reacts to annoyances and frustrations, just as yours does. If the home is not happy, if there are rows between the parents, if mother is preoccupied with other problems, then bowel training is slow.

44. Constipation in School-Age Children

Bowel habits acquired in babyhood continue in the preschooler and in the school-age child. By the time the toddler is ready for school, he should ideally be trained to use the bathroom at about the same time every day. That time should preferably be after a meal, so as to give his gastrocolic reflexes scope to act naturally. Additionally, the chosen time must not conflict with periods when everyone else in the home is clamoring to use the family bathroom, and it should not conflict with school activities.

The gastrocolic reflex is at its best after breakfast, but in a large family, if mother, brother, sister, and father in turn hammer at the bathroom door, then the most sensitive member of the family is bound to feel unwelcome there. This feeling of being resented when occupying the family throne in the mornings can become a subconscious conviction that the child is doing wrong when occupying the seat at any time.

In school there are additional problems. Teachers naturally do not care to see a continuous parade of children marching in and out of the classroom. They suspect, rightly so, in some instances, that dancing off to the bathroom is a variation of playing hookey. Also, kids are little horrors towards each other at times. They giggle and make snide remarks when one child puts up his hand too often. During intermissions the school bathroom becomes an extension of the playground and may become a battleground. Water faucets become ammunition dumps for the time-honored water-squirting fights. Sexual games are played in the school bathroom, too. No sooner does a child with a genuine need to sit on the toilet close the cubicle door, when someone starts peering underneath it, or over it. Children are naturally curious about sex. At certain stages of development, bowel function and sex are synonymous. Some children never grow out of that stage. They become the kind of adult who tells bathroom jokes and may even be prone to overt sexual perversions.

If your school-age child suffers from constipation, assign him the undisturbed use of the family bathroom at the same time every day. That time should preferably be after a meal, but if this is not possible, then another time of day will have to do. You will then be ignoring your child's gastrocolic reflexes, but if that is unavoidable then so be it. You then count on developing his visceral learning. It takes longer, but it works. Tell your child to sit on the throne for fifteen minutes every day. He or she can have something to read or can do his homework or can listen to a transistor. Tell him not to strain but to genuinely try. Reward him for success with understanding and a matter-of-fact smile of encouragement. Do not make a big thing out of it. Do not give him candy, material rewards, or money. Above all, encourage him to persevere. It takes a toddler two years to attain bowel control to the stage of regularity. If your child missed that stage originally, it will take him some time to catch up.

At the same time, see to it that your child's diet is not constipating. In practice this means cutting down on milk, increasing the amounts of fish and other high-protein foods and switching from white bread and cakes to wholemeal brown bread. A good idea is to give him some bran every day, either as bran cookies or sprinkled on sandwiches or breakfast cereals. Increase the amounts of fresh fruit and fresh tender vegetables you serve every day. Make him drink lots of fluids.

Use laxatives only as a last resort. *Before* you do, read the sections on laxatives in Part IV.

45. Emotional-Crisis Constipation

A sigmoidoscopy is the medical examination of the inside of the lower bowel through a tube-shaped instrument called a sigmoidoscope. There is a story about a doctor who was performing a sigmoidoscopy on a particularly shy male patient. The doctor was peering intently into the sigmoidoscope, when suddenly he saw the inside of the intestine blush. The doctor looked up. A particularly attractive nurse had just entered into the room. The patient's face was red, too. The nurse had noticed nothing.

The human bowel reacts to emotional upsets in various ways. Sometimes its response is nervous diarrhea, discussed in Section 17. At other times it responds with constipation.

Major crises that can cause acute constipation are a broken engagement, the loss of a job, a death in the family. The cause of the upset in children is sometimes not so obvious. I have seen it result from a fight between parents, the arrival of a baby brother, moving to a different city, and even changing from one school to another.

Major emotional crises unfortunately do occur. In some cases they can reach what psychologists call peak experiences, which then color a person's outlook, behavior, and bodily functions for the rest of life. When viewed in retrospect, peak experiences are not always deleterious. They may be beneficial.

The person afflicted with an emotional-crisis constipation is not likely to pay attention to it until it becomes extreme, when urgent relief becomes necessary. The best treatment is an enema, but a gravely upset individual is unlikely to bother with that. The next best remedy is a dose of salts, as described in Section 56.

In due time emotional-crisis constipation gives way to reactive diarrhea. There is a chance that the sufferer will then be tempted to treat the diarrhea with medicines, which on the rebound may lead to another bout of constipation. If the emotional crisis is still not resolved, then diarrhea and constipation alternate, in the pattern described in the sections on spastic colitis or the irritable bowel syndrome. (Section 48).

If you or someone else in your family should suffer from this kind of disability, do not just seek relief from your bowel problems. Seek professional help about the crisis.

46. Inactivity Constipation

Already described is the acute constipation followed by reactive diarrhea that is the lot of the traveler (Section 25). Constipation is apt to follow inactivity from any cause. The student who sits for days cramming for examinations is prone to it, and if luck is against him, the inevitable rebound diarrhea will be augmented by emotional causes and will hit him just at the time when he will be wishing that he could forget about his intestine—during his exam.

Inactivity constipation is the vexation of the person who sits at a desk all day and stares at a TV screen all evening. It plagues the astronaut in his space capsule and the senior citizen in his rocking chair. The more unaccustomed, the stricter, the more prolonged the immobility, the worse is the constipation. Hospitalized patients suffer from it so often that many doctors make it their habit to prescribe laxatives as part of their patients' hospital routine. Nurses are more than familiar with the problem. They would rather administer laxatives in time than have to give enemas.

Complete body immobilization, as in a hospital bed, is dangerous in many other ways, too. There is an ironical truism that "a bed is a dangerous place to be—most people die in bed." Immobilization in bed causes sluggishness of the circulation and a real risk of blood clotting in the veins. Such a blood clot can migrate, get stuck in the heart, and kill. Muscles waste from disuse, cause weakness. Lungs are not ventilated properly; there is a danger of pneumonia. Even bones become decalcified and brittle.

The cardinal part of the treatment of any ailment is prevention. Inactivity constipation should be prevented, not treated. If you are a student cramming for an examination, break your studying every hour or so. Go outside. Get a few lungsfull of air kicking a ball around, then return to your books. You will not only please your digestion but will retain more of what you are studying. If you work in an office, remember that chaining a person to a workbench went out with the passing of the galley slaves. Find some excuse to move around. Stretch your muscles. If nothing else works, make full use of such established office institutions as the washroom and the water cooler. Walk or bicycle to work. Do not try to park your car right outside your place of work. If you work in a factory, point out to your union representative that the Japanese are doing quite well, thank you, with a system under which all work in a plant stops for a calisthenics break every so often. Don't laugh—it could be done here, too.

In the evenings, don't just sit there glued to the idiot tube. Get up and do something. Get an active hobby. Join an active club. If everything else fails, get a dog. You will gain not only a true friend and a companion; you will also have a constant reminder to go for walks.

There are occasions when immobility is hard—but never impossible—to prevent. Astronauts in space set time aside for exercise. In hospitals, detailed routines specify that almost all patients must be out of bed and walking on the morning following operations. It hurts to move after undergoing surgery, but that is not important. Postoperative pain can be eased with drugs, and in any case, pain is not dangerous. Nobody dies of pain. Immobility is dangerous. You can die from immobility. I tell my own patients that I will put thumbtacks or fire-crackers or ants in their beds if they do not move. I have never done that to anyone . . . yet; but I have been tempted! When bedrest is necessary—for example, after some forms of heart attacks or in some spine injuries—a physiotherapist is detailed to get the patient to breathe deeply, to bend and stretch legs, to flex and work the bicepses, many times a day. Even that little exercise is better than none.

In the treatment of established inactivity constipation, one must distinguish between an acute constipation in a usually active person and a chronic constipation in the person who is habitually inactive for some reason. In the former, the best treatment is an enema; since this is not generally acceptable to most people, the next best is a dose of salts. A saline laxative has almost the same effect as an enema. It produces some cramps and some abdominal pains, and its effect is slower than an enema, but its action is reliable. The dose you take must be just right for you. Your own system may require a little more or a little less than the label says. If you take too little, you may end up with just cramps but no evacuation. If you take too much, the action may be too violent for comfort. Salts should be taken on retiring at night, when they will go "whoosh" first thing in the morning. For a description of the properties of different salt laxatives, see Section 56.

There are always other factors in the causation of constipation in people who are chronically inactive and chronically constipated. If you are one of those people, read the section on the treatment of habitual constipation and follow the instructions given there (Section 50).

47. Drug-Caused Constipation

Look long enough at TV drug commercials and you may be tempted to believe that there exists, right here on earth, a chemical heaven with pearly gates labeled "Fast, Fast, Fast Relief" and "Something for Nothing." On this side of Alice's Looking Glass, however, drugs are not that perfect. All have disadvantages as well as advantages. All are capable of producing their share of the side effects that were detailed in Section 23. Quite a few of them produce constipation.

Until 1962 drug manufacturers in the United States were not required to list the constituents of their products on container labels. Then came the thalidomide tragedy. Next came Ralph Nader and the pressure of consumer groups. Drug laws were tightened. Labeling regulations were made increasingly strict. At the time of writing, the latest amended federal food, drug, and cosmetic act and the regulations enforced by the Food and Drug Administration of the U.S. Department of Health, Education, and Welfare have abolished the patent medicine concept. In the United States, the consumer can look at the label of any over-the-counter drug and see exactly what he is buying. In Canada, patent medicines with "secret ingredients" unfortunately still exist. They are regulated by the Proprietary and Patent Medicines Act. Their ingredients are kept on file in poison-control centers in major hospitals. The well-established, better-selling brands are also listed in major compendiums of pharmacology such as the Martindale *Extra Pharmacopeia,** copies of which may be found in large libraries. To date, however, the Canadian consumer has no readily available information of what may lurk in the nostrums advertising is pushing on him.

There are three groups of widely used drugs that regularly produce constipation:

1. Pain relievers containing codeine (also, on prescription only, opium and morphine).
2. Cough and cold preparations containing codeine, dihydrocodeine, hydrocodone bitartrate, dihydrocodeinone bitartrate.
3. Almost all indigestion remedies and antacids—that is, preparations used in the treatment of acid indigestion, peptic duodenal and gastric ulcers, and gastritis, especially if they are mixed with the antispasmodic drugs derived from belladonna: atropine, hyoscine (scopolamine), and hyoscyamine.

If you are prone to constipation and if you live in the United States, look at the list of ingredients on the label of the pain, cold, cough, sinus, or indigestion remedy you are buying. Avoid those that feature any of these drugs among their ingredients.

In Canada, if you wonder if the "Fast, Fast, Fast" remedy will block your digestion, telephone your nearest poison control center, listed in the telephone book. Theoretically you can get the information for the asking.

You should have no trouble finding pain relievers and cough and cold remedies that do not contain codeine or its derivatives. Numerous alternatives exist, both on prescription and over the counter. You do not have to remember the long names, either. Notice that all the constipating ingredients share the word root "code." Simply avoid taking any pain, cough, and cold

* London: Pharmaceutical Press, 1973, 2,320 pp.

remedies that contain any ingredient with the word root "code" in it.

If you suffer from "acid indigestion," peptic ulcer, or gastritis, then your constipation problems are not solved so easily. There are no good antacids that do not also produce some constipation in some people. Moreover, your diet probably contains much milk. Excess milk has a binding effect on most people.

If you have to take antacids and as a result find yourself constipated, consult your doctor about taking an antacid preparation that has a mild laxative mixed in. Do not take such mixes without medical advice. Many proprietary antacid-laxative mixtures contain mineral oil and are not suitable for long-term use. (See the section on laxatives in Part IV this book.)

In most instances you can balance the constipating effect of antacids, and yet not compromise your ulcer diet, by taking separately one of the bulk-producing laxatives described in the section on laxatives. Again, do not do this without obtaining medical advice first.

48. The Irritable Colon

The word "spa" is somehow un-American, and definitely un-Canadian. The concept which it encompasses is foreign to our continent. It smacks of neurosis, of sinful self-indulgence, of dollars wasted, with no consumer goods to show in return.

Many a North American tourist would do well to

stop at any of the hundreds of spas of the old Continent. Not only stop and rubberneck, but stay for a while. One week is not enough. Two weeks is the minimum which frazzled nerves, and tense muscles, and spastic bowels need, to tune into the purposeful quiet which pervades these establishments. There is an unhurried elegance about a good spa; a singularity of purpose which cannot even be even grasped in less time. At least a second, two-weeks stay is necessary before the discipline hidden in the beautiful surroundings can take full hold, for, like Transcendental Meditation or the exercises of Yoga, successful spa treatment is something that must be learned.

Spa treatment consists of more, than just walking from one splashing fountain to another, sipping from a glass of sulphurous tasting water, and listening to an outdoor orchestra playing Mozart or Strauss. Thanks to the genius of the ancient Romans who invented it over 2,000 years ago, spa treatment is a method for attaining something that modern science until recently thought impossible: the acquisition of conscious control over one's subconscious tensions.

The disease variously known as the irritable colon syndrome, spastic colitis, and mucous colitis is an abnormal tension of the bowel, characterized by cramps and spasms that at times approach a constant spastic state. An obstinate constipation results. The infrequent stools are passed in small hard lumps like the stools of a deer or else in long narrow ribbons, called toothpaste stools. Bouts with explosive diarrhea alternate with the constipation if, as frequently happens, the individual resorts to laxatives. (These last two symptoms—change in the stools' diameter and alternating constipation and diarrhea—can also be a sign of colon cancer.) Emptying the bowel by this means does not, however, give relief. Even though the intestine may be empty, the sufferer continues to feel the urge to evacuate. On repeated trips to the bathroom, he suffers and strains but only passes mucus; hence the name mucous colitis.

Together with the disordered bowel function, the

patient also experiences severe abdominal cramps, amounting to fierce pain at times. Much gas is passed, together with belching—all to the tune of assorted squeaks, growls, and rumbles from the unhappy intestine, a condition known as meteorism.

People suffering from an irritable colon forever make the rounds of doctors' offices. They undergo endless expensive tests and x-ray examinations, which invariably show little or nothing wrong. They try this treatment or that. Every so often their symptom patterns suggest to doctors that they suffer from some acute conditions, such as appendicitis, gall bladder disease, bowel obstruction, or worse. As time marches on, their bellies become criss-crossed with scars from operations. Some of them become addicted to painkilling drugs. In between they are told that they suffer from "nerves" or from hypochondria, or they are suspected of malingering. It is not a pleasant disease!

The typical patient suffering from an irritable colon is an unhappy, tense individual who must expend a fantastic amount of willpower to control his emotions. He eats too fast, and gets involved in all kinds of troubles at work, at politics, and at play. He is often highly intelligent but lacks insight into the nature of his disability. He works too hard, sleeps too little, and worries because his colitis interferes with his job. The worry makes his colon perform even worse. The worse his abdomen feels, the more he worries. This, in turn, makes him strive for ever more perfection in all his endeavors, yet success does not bring him the satisfaction he feels he deserves.

If you are such an individual, you must first and foremost recognize that you have a disability, much in the same way as a person who suffers from diabetes or has lost an arm or a leg. This may seem easy advice to give, but no other counsel will do any good. You absolutely must come to terms with your disability. To have an unruly colon is not the end of the world. There are people who suffer from terrible headaches. There are people who are blind or deaf or confined to wheelchairs, yet lead happy, productive lives. In comparison to these tragedies, an irritable colon is a light cross to bear. It may help you to read biographies of famous people, to see how others have managed to overcome their handicaps. If you succeed in adjusting to your problem, then your bowel irritability will improve.

Second, your doctor can help you by prescribing a sedative or a tranquilizer, but do not expect too much from the drug. Neither your doctor nor the tranquilizer can change your basic attitudes or outlooks. You yourself must do it. You can do it by an act of continuous autosuggestion or self-hypnosis or, if you prefer to call it thus, by an act of will.

Lead an ordered, regulated life. This means that you should avoid jobs that are too taxing and love affairs that are too stimulating. Realize that there are limits to what you can do. There was only one Albert Einstein, one Casanova, and one Abraham Lincoln. All the other scientists and lovers and politicians in this world had to be content with less. Leave the gambling and the chance taking to others.

Third, watch your diet. Read the sections in this book that deal with diet in constipation. See to it that your diet is rich in roughage. This is important. You want your overactive peristalsis to be able to get a grip on something substantial, not to have it go into contortions trying to propel liquids. Eat only wholemeal bread. Avoid all baked goods made of white flour. Eat extra vegetables and tender fresh fruit. On your breakfast table, beside the sugar bowl, always keep a bowl of bran. If your supermarket does not stock bran, buy it from a health food store. It only costs pennies. By itself, bran tastes like horse fodder. Sprinkle a generous teaspoon or two of bran on your breakfast cereal. This will mask its taste somewhat. If you like brown bread with butter and jam, sprinkle a teaspoon of it on top of the jam. This way it actually tastes good. Find ways to add bran to all home baking.

Fourth, if you have a chance to do so, by all means

weeks each year at some spa. It's a great e a vacation.

the spa prepared to enter into the spirit of the establishment. See a spa physician, who will examine you thoroughly, review your x-rays and laboratory tests, then will prescribe exactly how many glasses of the foul-tasting water you should drink while promenading for so many miles among the bronze and marble statuary, over sunlit loggias and under shade dappled pergolas, pausing at limpid pools where carp fight for scraps of bread, and gazing at crystal streams tumbling over rocks. This will be your daily exercise. The physician will also prescribe for you exactly how often and for how long you should rest on a deckchair between your walks, and will tell you whether you should swim in the azure swimming pools or sweat it out immersed in packs of hot mud. The stay will charge your batteries. You will return home improved.

Finally, read the section on laxatives and enemas in Part IV. Avoid the stimulant and the irritant laxatives like a plague. If you must take something, stick to bulk producers and softeners, and don't be adverse to giving yourself an occasional enema if things become bad.

49. Diverticulosis, Diverticulitis

The *Oxford Universal Dictionary* defines the word "diverticulum" as "a smaller side-branch of any cavity or passage." In late medieval literature the word had a more sinister meaning: it was used to describe a hidden cul-de-sac or ambush where troublemakers were apt to congregate. In medical usage both definitions apply equally well.

Diverticula of the bowel are little outpouchings, or hernias, usually about the size of a pea, scattered about the lower colon. The condition of having diverticula is called diverticulosis.

Diverticulosis occurs in over 40 percent of all middle age and older people living in the Western world. As is the case with many forms of heart disease and gall bladder disease, if you live all your life in Africa or Asia, you run a good risk of dying of hunger, but you will not develop diverticulosis. Living here, if you are forty-five or older, chances are four in ten that you have it.

Until quite recently the cause of diverticulosis was a mystery. Today, thanks to the researches of men like Dr. Neil Painter of London, England, we do know how it is produced. Thanks to Dr. T. L. Cleave, also of En-

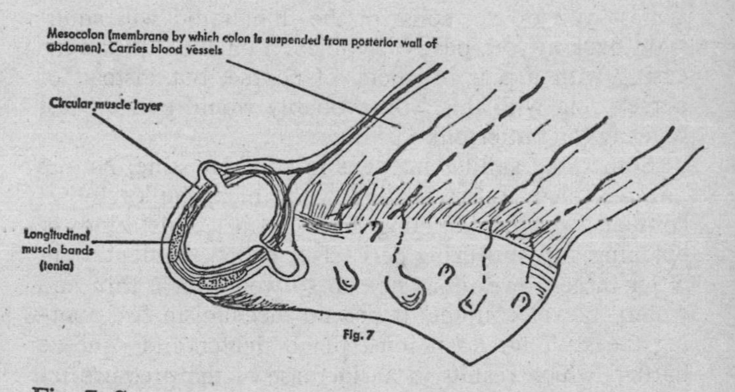

Fig. 7. Segment of colon showing diverticulosis.

gland, we know how to prevent it and how to treat it.

The condition diverticulosis, and its complication diverticulitis are two of the many items of tribute you pay for the privilege of enjoying highly refined foods. It happens this way:

As was described in Section 32, the food mash in your intestine does not just flow passively through your bowel but is pumped onward by a squeezing action of your intestinal muscles called peristalsis. Of the several forms of peristaltic action, the one that interests us now is the phase of segmentation.

Imagine, if you will, that you are stuffing a long sausage casing with sausage meat. You have managed to push so much meat into the open end of the sausage casing. You then pinch off the casing at the opening. Next, you squeeze the segment of the casing beyond the place where you have pinched it. This propels the meat onward. To get the meat still farther along, you pinch the casing again. Once more, you squeeze. And so on.

Now imagine that, instead of using sausage meat, you try to fill the sausage casing with a thin, liquid substance, say, buttermilk. Right away you notice that the pinching and squeezing technique does not work so well. You have to pinch tighter and squeeze harder. Unless you do so, some of the thin liquid will squirt right back at you, past your pinch. You could pinch the casing with a pair of pliers, of course, but instead of persevering with this, you probably would end up just pouring the buttermilk in.

Something similar happens in your intestine. Nature has designed it for dealing with thick, bulky bowel contents, propelled along best by just this kind of pinching and squeezing peristalsis, called segmentation. Your large bowel does not do so well with a thin and watery bowel content. It has no mechanism for pouring the stuff in. So it must pinch tighter and squeeze harder, which results in an increase of the pressure inside the bowel. The bowel wall becomes overstressed. As the years go by, the continued overpressure weakens the muscle layer of the bowel wall and causes tiny splits in it. The soft inner layer of the bowel bulges and blisters through these splits, much as an overinflated inner tube eventually bulges and blisters through defects in the casing of a tire.

The cause of diverticulosis is a diet that lacks sufficient residue for easy and efficient segmentation peristalsis. This is the type of diet enjoyed in North America. Its main culprits are white flour used in the baking of bread, cookies, cakes, and so on, and refined sugar. Also important is the omission of enough fruit and vegetables. The longer you have eaten refined flour goods and refined sugar, and the more you have liked to eat these things over the years, the higher is the chance that you now have diverticulosis.

There is a link between diverticulosis and the irritable colon problems described in the preceding section. In spastic colitis (irritable colon) the pressure gradients in the large intestine are increased. People who suffer from colon spasticity are more prone to develop diverticulosis. Although established, noninflamed diverticula are not painful and do not need any treatment, *diverticula in the making* are a source of pain. The pain comes partly from the bowel spasms, partly from the splitting of the muscular casing of the intestine and the blistering of the diverticula through the splits. This stage of the illness cannot be seen on an x-ray examination, which only shows already formed diverticula, but it nevertheless has a name. The name of this stage, appropriately enough, is painful diverticulosis, or spastic diverticulosis.

Once diverticula are established, your body hastens to surround them with bolsters of fat. If you watch your diet and all goes well, your fully established diverticulosis will not give you a moment's trouble, even if you live to the age of 150. If you are unlucky, fecal material will get trapped in some diverticula and irritate them, and the bacteria within them will cause an infection—much like what can also happen in your appendix. This complication is called diverticulitis.

Diverticulitis is largely preventable. If you mend

your dietary ways, chances are that you will never suffer from it. It is an acute disease that comes on quickly and shows itself by pain, usually on the left side of the abdomen. Many cases are mild. Some clear up with no treatment. It can, however, be as severe as appendicitis and result in abscess formation and perforation. It can also become chronic, with repeated attacks. It should be treated by a doctor.

Segmentation Pain

Segmentation spasm, which causes a high pressure gradient in a portion of the intestine, gives trouble in other ways, too. It is the cause of otherwise unexplained belly aches and even acute pains. In the case of young people, especially girls, it can give rise to a fierce discomfort in the right lower side of the abdomen, in the portion of the colon called the cecum. A valve mechanism at the junction of the small bowel (ileum) and the cecum can, if shut from spasm, completely eliminate any chance of the pressure build-up relieving itself back in the direction of the small bowel. The resultant violent pain mimics appendicitis. The high pressure can *cause* appendicitis. Many people have lost their appendices because of this condition—rightly so, because a doctor cannot be sure which of the two it is and removing the appendix is safer than leaving it. Problems arise again, when pain recurs after the appendix has been removed. Many a woman has been told that this pain comes from her ovary or from an infection of her tubes.

Adults and middle-aged and older people suffer from this kind of pain a little higher up, on the right side. Here, the worrisome organ is the gall bladder. If the gall bladder contains stones, it should come out. If it does not contain stones or if the pain persists after the gall bladder has been removed by operation, chances are high that the pain is due to colon segmentation spasm. It can, however, be due to other causes.

Do not neglect abdominal pain. Do not just assume that it is due to segmentation spasm. Do not treat it with laxatives or with any medications. Consult your doctor about it.

Prevention and Treatment

Until quite recently the standard medical advice to sufferers from diverticular disease was to eat precisely the kind of low-residue diet that produced the disease in the first place. There was no understanding of the true cause of the illness. Doctors vaguely supposed that the indigestible residue of the diet had something to do with it, that excessive residue somehow punched the diverticula out, and that more residue would just get jammed into them, would distend them, would cause infections, and so on. Patients did not improve but it was supposed that the disease was progressive in spite of the diet advice. Old beliefs die slowly.

To avoid developing diverticulosis and its complications, eat as little of highly refined white flour foods and refined sugar foods as your taste buds allow. Stick to wholegrain bread. Avoid gooey cakes and sugary cookies. Avoid drinking excessive amounts of sugary soft drinks. Eat more fresh and tender green vegetables and fruit. Eat some bran every day.

Bran is by far the best sort of roughage in these cases. Since it is a dried product of ripe grains, it would seem to be, by the definition stated in Section 35, to be an "undesirable" kind of roughage. Bran is an exception. Its particle sizes are small—quite unlike the long fibers of overripe fruit skins, tough vegetable leaves, and woody stalks, which tend to bind constipated stools together, like so many iron rods used to reinforce concrete. In addition, bran has the property of swelling by absorbing water. It thus not only is a source of roughage but also acts as a bulk-producing laxative (see Section 54). Unprocessed bran is not exactly palatable, but it does not taste badly when mixed with breakfast cereals, and it actually improves the taste of syrups and jams. In addition, it can be mixed into soups and stews. Its constipation-preventing action is remarkable. Dr. T. L. Cleave proved this when he ordered it to be placed on the mess tables of the thousands of sailors who manned the British battleship *King George V*. The crew of a warship on long patrols during World War II did not often get the chance to eat fresh fruit or vegetables or to indulge in much exercise. Bran kept those sailors "going." It will do the same for you.

There is one laxative that can occasionally be tried, strictly under a doctor's supervision, and only in cases of proven spastic diverticulosis. This laxative is castor oil. It seems to act by overcoming spasm and clearing the diverticula. It can give relief from pain, sometimes for prolonged periods. Its use in cases of undiagnosed abdominal pain is dangerous. It can blow out an appendix, cause peritonitis. It can do other harm. Never use laxatives in abdominal pain unless advised to do so by your doctor.

If your diverticulosis ever deteriorates into diverticulitis, the diet advice is different. In this disease—and a disease this is, not a "condition"—the old-fashioned advice of low-residue or no-residue diet still applies. If you should suffer a bout of diverticulitis, drink only clear liquids. This excludes milk. Now you want your bowel to be empty, to let the inflammation subside, to let any pus in the diverticula drain into the bowel. Do not try to treat a bout of diverticulitis yourself. This is a job for your doctor. He will advise you in detail about what constitutes a low-residue or no-residue diet and will also prescribe for you drugs that will quieten, paralyze in effect, the violent peristaltic movements the liquid diet will cause. The best drug available at the time of this writing is propanthelidine bromide. It is a potent drug, capable of producing many alarming side effects. Do not take it on your own.

50. Chronic or Habitual Constipation

> "Who are *you*?" said the Caterpillar. This was not an encouraging opening for a conversation. Alice replied, rather shyly, "I—I hardly know, Sir, just at present—at least I knew who I *was* when I got up this morning, but I think I must have been changed several times since then."
>
> from *Alice in Wonderland*
> by Lewis Carroll.

I do not know why some people—many people—suffer from habitual constipation. I do know—or think that I know—that your bowel function is just one part of the very unique, never before existent, never again exactly reproducible entity that happens to be you. I can recognize certain factors that have molded your body and character, and your bowel habits. But beyond all this, beyond evolution, heredity, and environment, there is something else. This something used to be called human nature and even free will, in the days before the behaviorists held sway. Now that the behavior manipulators seem to be bowing out, this third force in you is once more a mystery.

Habitual constipation is in part due to inborn causes, in part due to the factors that have been discussed already. You may have been born with a less than perfect bowel. Your early toilet training may have been defective. Your childhood experiences at home and at school may have something to do with it. Emotional crises may have left their mark on you. Perhaps you do

.ot take enough exercise. It may be that you do not drink enough water. Your nervous system may be protecting your psyche from something worse, by afflicting you like this. You may be taking constipating drugs. You may be brainwashed by TV commercials into believing in laxatives and be addicted to laxatives. You may be suffering from various degrees of bowel spasticity. Above all, your diet has probably a lot to do with it.

Read through the sections dealing with different aspects of constipation with a pencil in your hand. Tick off and underline everything that applies in your case. Then summarize your findings and draw your conclusions. Then do something about it.

Read also the section on laxatives. Stay away from addicting laxatives. If you must take something, stick to the bulk producers and lubricants, and do not disdain the occasional enema. Get into the habit of eating enough of the right kind of roughage, and take some bran every day. Make full use of your gastrocolic reflexes. If your bowel has forgotten about them, train it anew. Set aside a time for sitting on the throne for ten to fifteen minutes, every day. Do not push or strain, but genuinely try. Don't become discouraged if you do not get results overnight. The term "habitual constipation" implies many years of misery. It may take a little time to retrain your intestines, but the small effort this takes will be worth it in the end.

51. Intestinal Function in Old Age

Have you ever noticed that time does not pass evenly? That clocks and calendars are liars? Have you given thought to the fact that a year in childhood lasts much longer than a year in middle age? And that, as the leaves of life turn gold, the hands on the clocks speed up until they race around the dials at dizzying speeds?

Don't let anyone tell you that it isn't so, that it only seems so. There are many ways of measuring time. The speed-up of your life is real. Let the clock face be a sign of warning to you: the less interest you take in life, the faster will your life end. When the fifth age of the Bard,* "in fair round belly, with good capon lined," is upon you, watch out. That fifth age is deadly! The obese, middle-age citizen "full of wise saws and modern instances," who habitually overeats, takes no delight in new things, does not exercise, and becomes constipated, is in great danger of dying from heart and blood vessel disease. Only the active and the slim can slow down the hands on the clocks and go onward to the sixth age, which "shifts into the lean and the slipper'd pantaloon, with spectacles on nose and pouch on side."

* The quotations in this section are from William Shakespeare's *As You Like It.*

To retire is easy. To enjoy retirement takes planning

and action. That sixth age can go on for a long time. I know oldsters in their nineties, who are still in it—people who have learned to cope with the physical disabilities and financial problems that old age brings and have discovered that there are also compensations. If your income now is smaller, so hopefully are your needs. You can look upon the foibles and the troubles of this silly world with the detachment they deserve. And even if your joints creak and your hands shake and you do get winded easily, take a little consolation in the knowledge that there are no diseases of the intestinal tract that are in any way whatever due to wear and tear or to growing old.

This does not mean, however, that your bowel function will now automatically improve. Any bad habits you have acquired earlier are liable to plague you still. But now you should use some of your newfound leisure to rectify them. If you have suffered from spastic colitis before, now is the time to attend to it. If you are a victim of chronic constipation, now is your opportunity to get rid of it.

Happy indeed is the person who continues to be curious, to be a doer, through the years. To such people will come the blessing of growing gradually more forgetful, more restricted mentally, until they slip into "the last scene of all, that ends this strange eventful history, the second childishness and mere oblivion, sans teeth, sans eyes, sans taste, sans everything." People who are scared of growing old themselves, yet who dread equally the thought of death, pity such a fate. It is not a pleasant prospect, yet of all the ways of departing from this world, this is one of the kindest. As awareness of surroundings slips away, so do the worries, the pangs of disabilities, the throes of sufferings. The senile individual has come to the end of the role he has played through a lifetime of influencing those who have lived alongside him and those who will follow him. Do not begrudge him the nursing care he now needs.

In the age of "second childishness and mere oblivion" bowel function becomes a real, though not an insoluble, problem. As in the case of the baby, this once again is the age of bowel incontinence. There are two types: incontinence due to inactivity, which leads to extreme constipation with overflow, and incontinence due to lack of central brain inhibition.

Inactivity constipation has already been described (Section 46). In the case of disabled, bedridden senile patients, the inactivity is apt to be total. Professor Brocklehurst of the University of South Manchester has demonstrated by the use of x-rays and x-ray opaque markers ingested by patients that in these circumstances the normal average twenty-three hours food transit time through the intestinal tract can increase to seven days. Since the primary function of the colon is to extract water from food residue, and consequently since the longer the stool stays in the colon the drier and harder it becomes, it is small wonder that totally immobilized people are apt to suffer from a constipation, in which the stools can become as hard as cement. Complete bowel obstruction due to this can, and sometimes does, occur. More frequently, the hard, cement-like mass forms a ball that sits firmly just above the anus. It can be the size of a football. Liquid stools find their way around it and over it, and percolate steadily through the anus. The result is a near constant soiling of the bedclothes. The same, it will be recalled, can also happen in small children (Section 30).

To prevent this condition, do not allow total immobility, even if the patient is paralyzed. He or she must be turned from side to side every few hours, must be sat up, must, if possible, be placed in a chair, must be moved around. Any such efforts on the part of relatives or nursing staff reflexly produce muscular responses on the part of the patient. Even the slightest activity makes a difference, and the more of it, the better. Besides prevention of impaction, such nursing care also prevents bed sores, bladder infections, contractures, and pneumonia.

Once the condition is established, the impacted ball

must be removed manually. This is not a pleasant job. Life is full of unpleasant jobs made necessary by the neglect of other jobs that should have been done on time. The nurse, orderly, or doctor must don a rubber glove, insert one or two fingers in the rectum, break up the bolus into pieces, then extract the pieces. Repeated enemas must then be given to complete the evacuation. The task can be lengthy; a very badly established impaction can take a week of twice-daily enemas to clear. The enemas should be of ordinary tap water slightly warmed. Saline enemas made up by adding three quarters of a teaspoon of kitchen salt to a quart of water are better still. Soap suds should not be used. They are shocking to a feeble patient and may be downright dangerous.

Further daily management must include adjustment of the diet with fresh fruit and juices and fresh, tender, green vegetables, as was detailed in the sections on diet. Two ounces of prune juice twice daily will help, as will the regular use of bran and perhaps also of a commercial bulk-producing agent, such as Metamucil (Searle), in doses of a teaspoon, two or three times daily, in orange juice. Milk and milk products should be limited. Finally, if all this is still not enough to prevent a recurrence, a bisacodyl type of commercial stool softener laxative can be given either every other day or three times a week, as well as an enema about once weekly. Most important, someone who cares must observe the patient carefully or be prepared to perform a rectal examination with a gloved finger often enough so that the impaction does not recur.

In the second type of senile bowel incontinence, the pertinent parts of the brain are no longer able to recognize reflex nerve signals telegraphed to it from a distended colon. The remainder of the brain may still function well, and the oldster could still be enjoying life but for the misery that he or she just does not feel the urge to evacuate. Consequently the restraining brain signals to hold motions back until the act of evacuation is socially acceptable on the toilet seat is also missing.

Accidents happen; first occasionally, then constantly. Bowel function becomes automatic. Movements occur as soon as the pressure of a mass of stool in the rectum becomes great enough to trigger a contraction of the lower colon. The act of movement of the bowels thus becomes a reflex relayed by the spinal cord; the brain is not consulted.

The management of such a patient is entirely different from that of the oldster who suffers from inactivity constipation but is again a matter of good nursing. Such a patient's colon still works perfectly. As was described in Section 32, the normal colonic mass peristalsis still occurs twice or three times daily. The gastrocolic reflexes are still active after eating. Thus, about all that needs to be done in most cases is to remind the oldster to sit on the throne at the appointed hour each day—much in the same manner as one does in toilet training a child in regularity.

The diet in such a case should be mildly constipating. Excessive amounts of fresh fruit and green vegetables must be avoided. Since this may result in a lack of vitamins, and since this in turn may lead to constipation, give your patient a multivitamin supplement daily. To help make the diet mildly constipating, include in it a sufficient amount of milk. Very helpful are small daily doses of a thick pudding made by mixing powdered skim milk with a little water. Add some flavoring agent to the mixture, such as vanilla or other extract. In really exceptional cases a very small daily dose of a simple kaolin and pectin antidiarrhea remedy can also be given.

Part IV. Laxatives, Purgatives, Cathartics, Enemas

52. Introduction

A Frenchman, talking about the elegance and artistry of his country's cuisine, once said that "you are what you eat." He was stretching a point, but his argument was sound. Everything you eat and drink—and, for that matter, everything you inhale, assimilate through the skin, or otherwise absorb—does indeed influence your body. That influence may be nutritious, stimulant, retardant, irritant, poisonous . . . or a bit of each. Even apparently innocuous substances produce effects through their bulk or frequency of ingestion or amount ingested, and so on. Eat one potato, and its effects are negligible. Eat potatoes daily, and they become for you a basic food. Eat only potatoes, and you will soon be sick. Eat too many potatoes at one sitting and you could die.

Laxatives, purgatives, and cathartics are substances that, when taken in certain amounts, on certain narrowly defined occasions, in the case of certain kinds of people, will produce the desired effect of emptying the lower intestinal tract. When they are taken for wrong reasons, on wrong occasions, in amounts either insufficient or excessive for age, body size, and body function, their action will prove unpredictable, unpleasant, or dangerous. Since most people buy and use laxatives without a doctor's prescription, it behooves them to know what a given dose, in a given situation, can reasonably be expected to do. Do not just listen to commercials, and do not be swayed by advertising. Thanks to Senators Durham, Humphrey, Nelson, and Kefauver, the United States federal laws direct that all non-prescription drugs must now list their ingredients on their labels. Canadian laws unfortunately do not, as yet, make this requirement, but the day of similar laws is hopefully coming. Learn to read the labels. The small print in which the generic names of drugs are printed is not that hard to read. The names themselves may be difficult to pronounce, but the small effort is worth it. Learn that aspirin is aspirin is aspirin, irrespective of whether it is called that, or any one of the sixty-eight (at last count) names under which it is marketed. Learn that in spite of the plethora of brands, there are, in reality, only a very few kinds of laxatives in common use today. Learn that you can not only avoid grief but also save money by knowing what are the active ingredients in those fancy packages.

By definition, laxatives are substances that have the effect of loosening the bowels; cathartics are a degree stronger; purgatives produce copious evacuations. Since the effects of nearly all of these substances (except for the bulk producers) is proportionate to the dose taken, the different designations do not mean much.

All laxatives can be divided into five categories. These are:

1. Natural laxatives
2. Bulk-producing agents
3. Softeners
4. Salts
5. Stimulants and irritants

IMPORTANT: All drugs, including all laxatives, are liable to cause trouble, even to the point of being dangerous, when taken for the wrong reasons; if improperly manufactured, impure, or deteriorated in storage; or else through the mechanisms of toxicity, cumulative toxicity, idiosyncrasy, intolerance, side ef-

fects, allergy, or withdrawal, which were described in Section 23. In this book I do not advise anyone to take any laxative or any other drug. The remarks that follow describe results that usually occur in the majority of people who use such drugs with due circumspection and prudence. I do not own a crystal ball and cannot predict how any one drug or any combination of drugs is likely to affect any one individual or group of individuals. NEVER take ANY laxative for abdominal pain. You could blow out your appendix, suffer a perforation of an obstructed bowel, and die.

53. Natural Laxatives

Natural laxatives are foods that make bowel motions soft and easy to pass. They have already been extensively dealt with in the sections of this book that deal with diet. Food items such as green, fresh, tender vegetables and slightly underripe fruit produce this effect because they contain chemicals that are slightly stimulant or irritant. In many cases the exact nature of these chemicals is not known. An exception is the chemical in prunes, a laxative principle called diphenyllisatin. A chemically similar principle is contained in dried figs. Malt extracts and brown sugar have actions that are almost identical. Since these are also easily digested, they are useful for adjusting the diet of babies.

Other foods are classified as natural laxatives because they contain high proportions of an indigestible residue. Again, many fruits and vegetables fall into this category. These also have been described already.

Still other vegetable substances not only are not digested but also absorb water and swell in the process. These are the bulk producers. The most important here are bakery goods made with wholegrain flour.

The normal person who eats a nourishing, balanced diet and does not suffer from diarrhea or constipation keeps his intestines happy, because the foods he eats contain the right proportions of all these items. He has no need to worry about vitamins or minerals either. A balanced diet supplies them automatically.

Eating the right foods is by far the best way to bowel health. Before you are tempted to buy something off a drugstore shelf, pause. Analyze your eating habits. Amend any shortcomings, first.

Brands:

Maltsupex (Abbott) contains a barley malt extract said to be a good source of carbohydrate for addition to babies' formulas and to unbalanced diets of adults.

Ovaltine (Ovaltine Food Products) is a beverage concentrate made from barley malt, cocoa, soy flour, skim and whole milk, with some vitamins and iron. As far as intestinal function is concerned, its milk contents tends to cancel out its malt.

54. Bulk-Producing Agents

Bran
Psyllium (plantago) seeds
Agar
Methyl cellulose
Carboxymethyl cellulose

Much of the contents of this book has dealt with bulk already. Bulk is necessary for the intestine to be able to get a grip on its contents in order to squeeze it along. Food roughage supplies most of the natural bulk. The exact amounts needed daily to maintain health are not known. Nutrition councils have, to date, ignored the question. A balanced diet will supply the necessary bulk.

Additional bulk is necessary whenever a person lives on highly refined precooked or prepackaged foods, on sugary foods, on TV dinners, or on trashy snacks. It is of great value in the treatment of habitual constipation due to inactivity and immobility. It is essential after many operations on the intestine and especially after operations on hemorrhoids.

Bran is discussed in Section 49. In addition to its other virtues, it has the great advantage of being cheap.

Psyllium (plantago) seed is the next most useful bulk-producing agent. The ground seeds soak up water (or fruit juice) rapidly, then swell to the consistency of gelatin. They are an excellent way to assure bulky, formed yet soft, stools. They produce no known side effects. Allergies to them occur but are rare. Single doses are not effective; they must be taken three times daily over several days, together with lots of fluids, before an improvement can be expected. The leading commercial brand available presently is expensive. Since the ground seeds interfere a bit with the intestinal absorption of bile salts, they may, when taken routinely, give an added bonus of a modest reduction in the level of serum cholesterol.

Agar is a dried, gelatinous substance made of seaweed. Its action is similar to psyllium's. It, too, is a very satisfactory bulk-producing agent for routine use, but for some (unknown to me) reason it is not as widely used here as in other countries. A soft, formed stool is evacuated after its use in about eight to twelve hours.

Methyl cellulose, carboxymethyl cellulose, and other chemically allied cellulose compounds produce results that are similar. They absorb water, swell, and become gelatinous. They are poorly, if at all, assimilated from the digestive tract and serve to produce stools that are bulky, soft, and easy to pass. Single doses are not effective; consequently they are of no use in acute constipation but are a very satisfactory adjunct in the treatment of chronic constipation, after operations, and so on.

Brands:

Unprocessed bran is available from food stores and health food stores. This is the best. *Processed bran* is an ingredient of many breakfast cereals, bran cakes, bran muffins, all-bran bread, etc.

Metamucil (Searle) is probably the most widely used bulk-producing laxative sold in North America. It is said to be a psyllium hydrophilic muciloid mixed with dextrose (a sugar). It is an excellent product but is expensive. People who suffer from diabetes should keep in mind that it does contain sugar. It is also available in even more expensive, prepackaged single doses in which it is mixed with a flavoring agent and with other ingredients that make it effervescent. These ingredients include sodium bicarbonate, which make them unsuitable for use by people on sodium-restricted diets. Other than taste, the effervescent form has no advantages over the dry powder.

Konsyl (Burton, Parsons Co.) is said to be prepared from the outer, musilaginous layers of ispaghula (blond, or Indian psyllium seed). It is not as popular as Metamucil, perhaps because the company that makes it has a smaller advertising budget. *Vi-Sibilin* (Parke-Davis) is said to be a water-absorbent preparation of psyllium (plantago) seeds with thiamine hydrochloride (vitamin B_1).

55. Stool Softeners

Mineral oil
DSS (dioctyl sodium sulfosuccinate)
DCS (dioctyl calcium sulfosuccinate)

The best-known and most widely used stool softener is *mineral oil.* It is a good remedy. It is cheap and it works. It does, however, have disadvantages. Since very little of it is absorbed from the intestine, too large amounts or too frequent dosages result in its oozing right through the intestinal tract and out of the anus. The upshot is an unpleasant, involuntary soiling of the underwear.

Mineral oil should never be used for prolonged

periods. It is not only a stool softener but also a lubricant. Like motor oil in an engine, it coats the whole of the intestinal lining with an oily film. This film interferes with the intestinal absorption of certain food items, notably vitamins A, D and K. A lack of these vitamins can be dangerous and can lead to illness, especially to an increased tendency to bleed after injuries.

Other than being oily, mineral oil has no taste. Consequently, quite a few people find it nauseating. If a person who has just taken a dose of the oil gags, then gasps for breath, some of it can go down "the wrong way" and find its way to the lungs. In the lungs the mineral oil can produce pneumonia.

For the benefit of travelers, mineral oil is known as liquid paraffin in England, *huile de vaseline* in France, *Vaselinöl* in Germany, and *oleum vaselini* in Italy.

Better than mineral oil are the softeners *DDS* and *DCS* (dioctyl sodium sulfosuccinate and dioctyl calcium sulfosuccinate). They are not oily and do not interfere with vitamin absorption. They are easier to take and do not tend to leak out of the rectum. They work by lowering the surface tension of water. They thus not only lubricate the intestinal passage but are also able to penetrate right into hard, almost dried-out stools and to soften them not only on the surface but also from within. Both DSS and DCS can, at times, cause crampy abdominal pain.

Both DSS and DCS have similar actions, so if you must take them, buy whichever brand of either of them is the cheapest. People who suffer from congestive heart disease, however, who are on a low-sodium (low-salt) diet, are better off taking the calcium compound (DCS).

Brands:

Mineral oil is usually sold unbranded. One exception is *Nujol* (Plough). Many combination laxatives are based on mineral oil. *Agarol* (Warner) is said to consist of 27.8 percent mineral oil with 1.32 percent phenolphthalein (a stimulant), and agar (a bulk producer). *Magnolax* (Wampole is said to contain in each ml.: 0.25 ml. mineral oil and 60 mg. magnesium hydroxide (a salt laxative, with glycerine and vanillin. *Petrolagar Emulsion Blue Label* (Wyeth) is said to contain 7 percent liquid and 13 percent light liquid paraffin; *Red Label* in addition, is said to contain 0.35 percent phenolphthalein (a stimulant).

Colace (Mead Johnson) is said to contain pure DDS.

Surfac (Hoechst) is said to consist of pure DCS.

Mixtures: *Gentlax DDS* (Purdue Frederick) is said to contain DSS and senna (an irritant). *Peri-Colace* (Mead Johnson) is said to contain DDS and cascara (another irritant). *Senokap* (Purdue Frederick is another mixture that is said to contain DSS and senna (an irritant).

56. The Salts

Magnesium sulfate (Epsom salts)
Magnesium hydroxide (milk of magnesia)
Magnesium oxide
Magnesium citrate
Sodium phosphate
Sodium sulfate (Glauber's salts)
Potassium sodium tartrate (Seidlitz powders, Rochelle salts)
Potassium phosphate
All spa waters
All laxative mineral waters

In full doses the laxative salts are considerably more powerful than either the bulk-producing agents or the stool softeners. To be effective, they must be taken dissolved in water—the more water drunk with them, the better. Not only are salts poorly absorbed from the intestinal tract, but by a peculiar physical phenomenon called hypertonicity, they interfere with the normal function of the colon of absorption of water. The net effect of this is that most of the water drunk with the salts goes through the entire intestine to be evacuated together with the stools, which are softened, broken up, and made watery in the process.

Salt laxatives thus have an action not unlike that of an enema, which is water—or a laxative salt solution—instilled into the bowel from below.

If an insufficient amount of water is taken with the salts, then another of their chemical peculiarities comes into effect. This one is called osmosis. It consists of an actual withdrawal of water from the body into the intestine, where it produces the effect of a watery stool.

The different salts vary in potency, speed of action, taste, and price. The gentlest of the group is usually considered to be magnesium hydroxide (milk of magnesia). The most potent is probably magnesium sulfate (Epsom salts), which produces a number of watery stools, together with abdominal cramps and pains, in three to six hours. In no cases is the speed of action or the number of stools exactly predictable. Taste is a matter of individual preference: sodium sulfate (Glauber's salts) has the worst reputation; magnesium citrate and potassium sodium tartrate (Rochelle salts) are considered pleasant tasting. The latter two also cost more. The most expensive of the laxative salts are natural mineral waters imported in bottles from the springs of the world's famous spas, such as Vichy water and Karlsbad water.

There are a very large number of commercially prepared, proprietary salts. Usually these are mixtures. Often these are elegantly compounded with bicarbonate of soda and citric acid so that they fizz or effervesce when water is added to them. Examples are Kruschen salts and Andrews salts.

Like all medicines, salt laxatives have advantages and disadvantages. They can be invaluable when used with discretion and with a knowlege of what they can and cannot do. If abused, they can cause disaster. First, the advantages: They are mostly pleasant to take, usually quick in action, reasonably reliable. Because they act much like enemas, they can empty an overfull bowel efficiently, with less straining (but often with more cramping pain) than the stimulant or the irritant laxatives. Following the use of salts, you should expect to have to do without another bowel movement for two to three days; it takes that long for a completely empty colon to fill again. That two-to three-day stoolless interval is *not* constipation. Do *not* treat it with another dose of salts.

Now the disadvantages: There are many. Magnesium salts can damage a person's kidneys; they should not be taken by anyone who has ever had any renal disease. Sodium salts are slightly absorbed; they should not be taken by anyone who suffers from heart disease and must stay on a low-sodium (low-salt) diet. The laxative effects of the salts are reasonably reliable but are not completely predictable. This means that rather large doses must be taken—with the consequence of cramps—because small doses may not act at all. More importantly, salt laxatives must not be taken frequently or routinely; because of their osmotic action they withdraw electrolytes from the body. If such a withdrawal takes place frequently, changes in the person's chemical balance will follow.

Anyone who suffers from hemorrhoids should know that the repeated passage of liquid stools is irritating. A dose of the salts can cause an attack of the piles.

Finally, adequate doses of salts almost always produce abdominal cramps and pains. The pain is caused by violent contractions of the intestine, which does its best to push along a watery bowel contents that does not offer any bulk for the intestinal peristalsis to get a grip on. This is unpleasant by itself, but it can also blow out an inflamed appendix or produce a twisting of the bowels or a number of other dangerous complications. This happens but rarely; however, if it happens to you, then the fact that it is a "rare" misadventure will be of no comfort whatsoever.

57. Stimulants and Irritants

Phenolphthalein
Bisacodyl
Castor oil
Cascara
Senna
Danthron
Other vegetable purgatives

Stimulant laxatives act directly on the bowel by a process of irritation. The irritated tissues are either the mucous membrane lining the bowel wall or the nerve endings in the bowel wall. In either case, the bowel responds with peristaltic contractions designed, as it were, to rid itself of the annoyance. It matters little whether one calls them stimulants or irritants; this depends on the dose taken and on the frequency of dosage. All bowel stimulants (irritants) are classed as purgatives. To get the same effects, some individuals must take up to four or in some cases eight times as much as others. This means that the occasional user cannot know if the average dose as recommended by the manufacturer on the package label will or will not work for him, or if in his particular case, his own bowel will perhaps respond with violence. All bowel irritants (stimulants) occasionally cause allergies, hypersensitivities, and side reactions. All can cause cramps, griping, and pain. Some of them are addictive. They do, however, work.

You may be already familiar with *phenolphthalein*, an indicator dye that changes color from clear to red when dripped into an alkaline solution. Its laxative career began in Hungary, in 1902, when it was investigated by the Hungarian government as a possible means of detecting adulterations of the country's excellent Tokay wines. It did not make the grade as a consumer protection agent for reasons that are now obvious, but it did succeed as a laxative. Thanks, in a large measure, to the advertising efforts of its principal manufacturer, the Ex-Lax Company, it is one of the most widely used purges today. In its pure form it is odorless and tasteless. It is effective in very small doses. It mixes well with chocolate. In distinction to, say, castor oil, taking it is no problem at all.

Phenolphthalein is a reliable remedy. It works. However, it too has disadvantages. It can produce allergic reactions—skin rashes, or worse. In addition there are two reasons why it should not be used routinely. First, the bowel gets used to being flogged by it and eventually will not, and cannot, empty itself without it. Phenolphthalein is addictive. Addicts to it never experience the sensation of well-being that comes from regular, natural, healthy bowel motions. Instead, they are awakened early each day with a feeling of desperate urgency. They rush to the bathroom, where their bowels go "whoosh." The sensation they are left with is one of temporary relief but also of fullness and anxiety and tension, which makes them take another dose again in the evening. After a few years of this kind of existence, the addict's anus can become so used to transmitting only liquids that it contracts and narrows by a process known as stenosis, until it can no longer accommodate normal-sized stools. Bowel obstruction by fecal impaction can follow.

The second reason why phenolphthalein should not be used routinely is shared by other stimulant (irritant) purgatives. Repeated, habitual, continual irritation of the lower bowel produces a chronic inflammation. This is not only unpleasant by itself but results in a constant outpouring of mucus, loss of the body chemicals called electrolytes, and a consequent chronic tiredness, chronic lassitude, chronic poor health.

A minor problem of phenolphthalein has been observed by people who have taken it by mouth, then for some reason have additionally taken a soap suds enema. Since soap suds are alkaline, the phenolphthalein colors them red. Unless a person is familiar with this peculiarity, he may think that the enema has made him bleed.

Bisacodyl has been in wide use only since 1953. Chemically it is related to phenolphthalein and its action is similar. It is an effective purgative. It is available both in tablet form and as suppositories for insertion into the rectum. It has been advertised especially as a "contact" laxative; the word "contact" means in this sense exactly the same as the words "stimulant" and "irritant" but sounds, I suppose, somehow better.

Bisacodyl has some modest advantages over phenolphthalein in that it does not color the stools or the urine red, and in that it is alleged to be less likely to produce allergic reactions. Since it can irritate the stomach and small intestine as well as the colon, tablets of it should not be chewed or crushed. As is the case in all stimulant purgatives, the dose effective for one person may be too big or too small for others; anyone contemplating its repeated use must find his optimal dose by trial and error. Cramping and griping pains and a "whoosh" type of response is to be expected if the dose is high. Bisacodyl suppositories are effective if the stool is not too dried out or impacted. The suppositories do, however, produce a burning sensation in the rectum.

Castor oil is a time-honored standby. It is one of the most reliable and also one of the fastest acting of the drastic purgatives. This is its main asset. Where other purgatives sometimes fail, castor oil almost always works.

Outside the body castor oil is a bland, soothing oil that is so innocuous that it can be used in eye drops and can be applied to the inflamed skin of a baby's bottom in the treatment of diaper rash. In the intestinal tract it is split chemically into acid substances that potently irritate the nerve endings of both the small and the large bowel. This attribute explains the rapidity of its action, as well as why it causes vomiting in some people.

The taste of castor oil is proverbially awful. There is no fear that it will ever be abused. Its main legitimate use is in the rapid cleaning out of the whole intestinal tract before x-ray examinations and before bowel surgery. To be effective it must be taken in full doses of at least one and a half or better still two ounces in the case of adults, proportionately less for children. This is important. Taking too little of it will cause much cramping and griping pain but no evacuation. Full doses produce repeated good evacuations, with relatively much less discomfort.

In the days when your grandmother was young, castor oil used to be a favorite remedy for the family's "Saturday night cleanout" routine. This misguided and cruel habit has now fortunately died out.

Cascara is made from the bark of the buckthorn tree. Its full name, *Cascara sagrada,* literally translated means "sacred bark." It is the most American of the purgatives. The white man learned about it from the Indians of California.

Being an irritant and a stimulant, cascara shares in most of the advantages and disadvantages of the other stimulants described. Although bitter in taste, it is more pleasant to take than castor oil. It is a reliable purgative that usually acts within six to eight hours. It is best taken on retiring, when it will produce one or more evacuations the following morning. The stool it produces is usually semisolid and not as violently "whooshy" and liquid as those produced by phenolphthalein or castor oil. It is a favorite ingredient of a great number of brand-name purgatives.

Senna acts similarly. It too is an ancient remedy. The West learned about it from the Arabs during the ninth century A.D. Like cascara and castor oil, it is an herbal remedy, obtained from the dried leaves of the cassia plant.

Highly purified extracts of senna are available and are called glycosides. They are marketed under several trade names. They are reputed to produce less cramping and less griping than the crude senna preparation. A thorough, usually single bowel evacuation within six hours can be expected after adequate doses.

Danthron is again similar in action. It may produce a pink discoloration of the urine and may temporarily stain mucous membranes brown. Neither of these side effects is serious, provided that the drug is taken only occasionally. Danthron can, however, appear in the milk of nursing mothers and give diarrhea to breast-fed children. Apart from these disadvantages it is a useful, albeit rather strong, purgative.

There remain a very large number of other vegetable purgatives, such as *aloes, rhubarb, ipomea, jalap, scammony, colocynth, gamboge,* and *elaterin.* All of these are either herbs or resins. All are too strong and too drastic in action to be used by themselves. They became obsolete when doctors forgot how to write compound prescriptions in which the effects of many constituents are delicately balanced against each other. The pharmacists of today no longer have the knowledge, or the time, to custom-mix the ingredients.

The old, almost-forgotten compounding formulas for these drugs read like poems of the heath or woodlands or like stories of the jungle. They call for leaves, barks, fruits, and roots to be lovingly gathered at just the right time of year; to be sorted, dried, pounded in a mortar with a pestle; mixed, infused with boiling water or saturated in alcoholic tinctures, then made up into individual pills on a pill board or else put up in sachets or prepared for use as teas. A few custom herbal supply houses still exist in England, on the old continents of Africa and Asia, even in North America, that have learned to mass market a pitifully meager number of these pharmaceutical works of art. I do not know enough about these drugs, or about the finished products, to hold a valid opinion about them. One example —Potter's Natural Herbal Tablets (Potter's Herbal Supply Co.), unobtainable in the United States—is said to contain aloes, cascara, dandelion root, fennel, holy thistle, lime flowers, myrrh, skullcap, and valerian.

The following obsolete purgatives are dangerous and should never be used: *calomel, podophyllum,* and *croton oil.* Calomel is a mercury compound that is downright poisonous. Podophyllum is so irritating that it blisters skin. Croton oil used to be used in the dark days of medicine for dosing chained victims of mental disease. It is so powerful that it is not fit to be given to an elephant.

Brands:

Most branded laxatives and purgatives of the irritant (stimulant) type are mixtures. The purpose of mixing or compounding several ingredients is to try to balance and bring out the most desirable feature of each. Since, in the case of purgatives, the actions of the various ingredients are not usually predictable on any one individual, the effects of mixtures are liable to be erratic and the incidence of allergies and side effects increased.

Ex-Lax (Ex-Lax) is said to consist of pure phenolphthalein in chocolate.

Dulcolax (Boehringer) is said to consist of pure bisacodyl and is also available in suppository form.

Kondremul with Phenolphthalein (Cooper) is said to contain phenolphthalein and mineral oil (a softener and lubricant). *Kondremul with Cascara* (Cooper) is said to contain mineral oil and cascara.

Dulcodos (Boehringer) is said to contain bisacodyl and DDS (a softener).

Peri-Colace (Mead Johnson) is said to contain cascara and DSS (a softener). *Glysennid* (Sandoz) is said to contain pure and native senna glycosides. *Gentlax DSS* (Purdue Frederick) is said to contain senna glycosides and DSS (a softener). *Darbane* (Riker) is said to contain pure danthron. *Darbantyl* (Riker) is said to contain danthron and DSS (a softener). *Doxidan* (Hoechst) is also said to contain danthron and DSS. *Senokot* (Purdue Frederick) is said to contain pure senna. *California syrup of figs* (Sterling) is said to contain senna, fig extract, ginger, oils of cassia (senna), peppermint, and cloves. *Innerclean* (Brooks and Warburton) is said to contain senna, frangula, psyllium, sassafras, buchu, agar, Irish moss, linum, and anise. *Carter's Pills* are said to contain phenolphthalein and aloes.

58. Which Laxative Is Best?

To the frequently asked question of which laxative is best, there is one answer only: there isn't one. First, it is better to avoid the use of laxatives altogether and to rely on diet, exercise, and all the other things described in this book. Next, although admittedly there are times and occasions when a laxative is needed by almost everyone, there is no one preparation or drug that is best for everybody, at all such times.

IMPORTANT: *Never use a laxative if you suffer from abdominal pain. Read the warning in Section 52. If you feel that you absolutely must do something to move your bowels while suffering from abdominal pa consult your doctor about the advisability of using a small saline enema. Even that carries an element of risk, but the risk of a small saline enema is less than that of an ill-advised purge.*

Small babies should never be dosed with laxatives. Adjust the diet as described in Section 38. If everything else fails, use a glycerine suppository.

Small children should very seldom require a laxative. Use a glycerine suppository, a small enema, or one-third to one-half of a bisacodyl suppository. In rare instances use milk of magnesia for acute constipation.

For older children use a suppository as outlined above, milk of magnesia, or a DSS softener. Avoid too frequent use of enemas for psychologic reasons; this may unduly focus the child's attention on his rectum and anus. Consult your doctor if you find that you are using any such medication frequently.

In cases of drug or food poisoning a full dose of one of the salts *given under a doctor's supervision* may be just the treatment to empty the intestine of the poison.

Before x-rays or before surgery on the intestinal tract there is nothing better and surer than a full dose of castor oil.

For people who should not strain because they suffer from a hernia or from heart disease, the laxative of choice is DSS or DCS. If this is not enough, then a DSS- or DCS-stimulant combination is indicated (for example, DSS with cascara or DSS with senna).

People who suffer from hemorrhoids and many other rectal diseases should aim at having soft, formed, but bulky stools. Their diet should be high in suitable roughage. They should eat extra bran and if necessary take a bulk-producing laxative, such as psyllium.

The constipation of sudden immobility is fully dealt with in Section 46. Its best emergency treatment is usually a dose of one of the laxative salts.

The treatment of the irritable colon syndrome is helped a great deal by a two- to three-week course of mild exercise combined with mental and emotional

a small daily dose of a mild saline
the essence of spa treatment. The kind
tive and its dosage should be individually
by a doctor.

onstipation of old age is described in Section 51. very case must be assessed individually. Enemas and bisacodyl suppositories can be given for the initial emptying of the bowel, followed by stool softeners such as DSS or DCS and bulk-producing agents such as bran and psyllium for routine follow-up use. If this is still not sufficient, then DSS-cascara or DSS-senna tablets can be resorted to, up to three times weekly.

59. Enemas and Suppositories

If anyone should think that flagpole sitting, telephone booth packing, marathon dancing, and streaking naked through crowds of people are particularly erratic fashions to which only recent generations are subject, let him read in the pages of the history of medicine. Read about the bloodletting fad to which the court of Louis XII was addicted, and read about the clyster (enema) frenzy that afflicted the court of Louis XIV. Read how the elegant and beautiful Madame Ninon de L'Enclos set the fashion of the day by having a small clyster administered to herself at least three times every day—and how the King himself, in one year, could withstand 47 bloodlettings, 212 purges, and 215 enemas, while being attended by no fewer than 107 doctors of assorted medical, surgical, iatromathematical, spagiristical (astrologico-alchemical), and botanical calling.

Times have changed. Today enemas are not the "in" thing at all. In fact, the mere thought of one is apt to strike the average citizen with apprehension if not disgust. In many ways this is good; overdoing anything is like squeezing an orange too hard—the initially sweet juice is apt to run bitter. But enemas still have a valuable place:

1. For the efficient, quick, and thorough evacuation of bowel contents (evacuant enema)
2. For administering specific medications to a diseased lower bowel (medicated, or retention, enema)
3. In exceptional cases, for administering water to a patient (hydration enema)

Since the lower bowel cannot absorb anything except water (and some few salts—see Section 2), the older concept of nutrient enemas is now obsolete.

Enemas are preferable to laxatives in that there are fewer dangers of allergies, sensitivities, drug intolerances, and so on. With their use, the diabetic need not worry lest they contain sugar, nor does the sufferer from heart disease need be concerned in case they contain sodium. They do not have to pass through twenty-odd feet of esophagus, stomach, and small intestine to reach the place where they perform their work; consequently they are not liable to cause nausea or vomiting. They act quickly—in minutes, rather than hours.

Both enemas and suppositories are infinitely safer to use in instances where constipation is accompanied by abdominal pain, which may or may not be due to appendicitis or other acute abdominal disease. (Even so, enemas can do harm in some of these cases, but are *much* less likely to do so than laxatives).

Enemas are wonderfully soothing before, and especially after, operations of all kinds.

What should you do if you have taken a dose of some laxative, now suffer from severe abdominal cramps, and it is obvious that the laxative has failed?

Do not take yet another dose of the same stuff. Do not now try another brand. Give yourself an enema.

Rectal suppositories serve similar purposes. They are small in bulk, do not require any paraphernalia for their administration, and are consequently easier to use. Some of them do produce a burning sensation in the rectum. Most can, infrequently, produce allergies. None is as efficient as an enema.

60. Classification of Evacuant Enemas

Bulk (or Wash-out) Enemas

The simplest enema is one of *ordinary tap water,* slightly warmed to body temperature. This is the best enema for home use. It will prove about as effective as most mixtures.

For small babies, for invalids, and for the very elderly use a *saline enema* prepared by dissolving about a teaspoon of ordinary kitchen salt in a quart (one milk bottle full) of slightly warmed tap water.

All other enemas combine the bulk or wash-out action of water with the chemical action of the substance dissolved in it. They have a slight advantage in that smaller amounts are necessary thus making them more comfortable to take and to retain. Their disadvantages are similar to those already described in the sections dealing with laxatives.

Softening Enemas

Softening enemas usually use *mineral oil* or a *mineral oil emulsion,* occasionally *mucilage* (a variety of starch). *Glycerine* in an enema acts partly as a softening agent, partly as a hypertonic solution to withdraw water from the system into the bowel by a process called osmosis, and partly as a mild irritant.

Irritant Enemas

These share some of the disadvantages of the irritant laxatives. The time-honored *soap suds enema* is homemade by swishing a cake of soap in warm water, until the water is slightly milky. Commercially made soap suds enemas consist of 2 percent to not more than 5 percent soft (liquid) soap in water. Spa enemas are eminently effective but can produce an acute inflammation of the bowel; they should not be used for babies or for people known to be suffering from any intestinal disorder or for the elderly. The *oxyphenisatin enema* is sometimes used in hospitals for thorough cleansing of the bowel before x-ray examinations. It is too powerful and too dangerous for home use.

Evacuant Suppositories

There are only two kinds of evacuant suppositories in common use. *Glycerine suppositories,* like glycerine enemas (see above), have a lubricant, hypertonic, and slightly irritant effect. They are suitable for use in babies and small children. They are not strong enough for reliable use in adults. Another item that can be used in babies is simply a sliver of soap held with the fingers for a short time in the baby's anus, where often it will produce the desired result then and there. A sliver of soap *must not be pushed in and must not be left in* a child's or anybody's rectum. *Bisacodyl suppositories* have been mentioned already in the section dealing with bisacodyl laxatives. They are suitable for use by adults. They work reasonably well if the constipation is not too severe, but they produce a burning sensation in the rectum, so any person with a rectal inflammatory disease is better off avoiding them.

Brands:

Water pollution notwithstanding, tap water still comes unbranded. Ordinary kitchen salt is sold under many brands—it does not matter which brand you use. Any good toilet soap will do for the preparation of a soap suds enema. *Travad 1500* (Travenol Laboratories) is a kit containing a plastic bag of 1500 ml. (53 fl. oz.) capacity, a length of plastic tubing, clamp, rectal tip, waterproof pad, funnel, and packet of soap. *The Fleet Enema* (Fleet) consists of a disposable, single-dose squeeze bottle that is said to contain 4 fl. oz. of a solution of sodium biphosphate and sodium phosphate. The same company also manufactures a disposable enema containing mineral oil. The products are convenient and satisfactory to use, except that the rectal tip of the squeeze bottles is too hard. *Lavema enema* (Winthrop) is said to contain oxyphenisatin.

Glycerine suppositories are sold under many brand names. *Dulcolax supositories* (Boehringer), *Laco suppositories* (Maney), and *Sopalax suppositories* (Pentagone) are each said to contain biscadoyl.

How to Give an Enema

For a baby or small child the best enema equipment is a small, all-rubber-bulb ear syringe. Since giving an enema to a child is apt to be messy, try to do it in the bathroom. If you must do it in bed, cover the bed first with sheets of newspapers, then with a waterproof piece of plastic, then with a towel. Don't forget to have a potty nearby. Lubricate the tip of the bulb syringe with petroleum jelly or any kind of face cream. Do not use soap. Have the required amount of slightly warmed enema solution ready in a container. If you are going to use tap water or saline, use up to 4 oz. for an infant, up to 8 oz. for a one-year-old, up to a pint for a five-year-old. Have the child lying on his left side or back. Gently insert the soft lubricated syringe tip into the anus. Slowly inject the required amount, refilling the syringe as necessary. Hold the child's buttocks together to prevent a premature—and messy—evacuation. Try not to inject any air. The less pressure you use and the slower you inject, the more effective the enema will be.

For an adult the time-honored equipment is a rubber hot water bottle with a length of rubber tubing attached. Better than that is a transparent plastic bag, where you can see at a glance how much of the enema solution has run in. The rubber or plastic tubing should have an efficient metal clip, with which you can shut off the flow with one hand. The tip of the enema outfit should be soft and ideally should be furnished with an opening directed slightly to one side. A urinary type catheter of the thickness of a ballpoint pen is best. Avoid enema tips that are pointed or hard or are made of metal.

First make up the required amount of the enema solution. If you are using tap water or saline, use 10 to 25 fl. oz.

The best room to use for the procedure is the bathroom. Have your patient lie on a bath towel on the floor, on his left side with his knees drawn up. Suspend the enema bag or can from a towel rail, not higher than two feet above the floor. Slide the soft, lubricated enema tip into the patient's anus about four inches. Then slowly, with frequent pauses, let the enema solution run in. Have your patient retain the solution for as long as possible (usually ten to fifteen minutes) before expelling it.

To take an enema yourself, the best place to do it is in a bathtub. Place a bath towel or bath mat in the empty bathtub. Have all your equipment ready. You can easily vary the pressure under which the enema solution flows in, by making up a hanger, with several hook-shaped bends on it, from a coat hanger. Suspend the coat hanger from the shower curtain rail; hang the enema bag from one of the bends in the wire, at a height that produces the most comfortable pressure at any given time—not over two feet.

Lie on the towel in the bathtub on your back or on your left side. Proceed to give yourself the enema in the manner that has been described already.

If you are using a glycerine, mineral oil, commercial salts, or soap suds enema, use the amounts recommended by its manufacturer.

Part V. Hemorrhoids

61. Introduction

Hemorrhoids are, in essence, varicose veins of the rectum. Like facial wrinkles and gray hair, they are so common that, if you do not already have them, chances are that you will. Now or in the future, when you do experience them, it is almost certain that you will find them embarrassing. Even today, when there are few taboos left, hemorrhoids are not a fit subject for polite conversation.

Some things you may have heard about their surgical treatment have perhaps amounted to horror stories. According to experts polled by—of all papers—*The Wall Street Journal,* only about 1 percent of all hemorrhoid sufferers submit to its "traditionally painful" surgery each year. The majority of sufferers prefer to treat themselves with nonprescription remedies, which at the time of writing sell across United States drugstore counters to the rustle of $40 million yearly.

That there is embarrassment about ailments of the most private parts of the human body is understandable. That this embarrassment results in widespread ignorance of one of the most important functions of the body is unfortunate. Ignorance leads to fear. Fear, in turn, is the root cause of unnecessary suffering. It is the predominant reason why the reputation of hemorrhoid surgery is so pernicious.

There is no mystery about hemorrhoids, and there should certainly be no fear about them. Their cause is inherent in the anatomic structure of the region of the body where they arise.

The rectum and anus are plentifully supplied with blood vessels. They have to be. They respectively hold, and transmit, the most infectious material that any region of the body has to deal with. The extensive network of arteries and veins about the rectum and anus serves to circulate infection-fighting blood freely through this tissue.

Arteries carry blood to this area under arterial blood pressure. Veins drain the blood back in the direction of the hydraulic ram that is the heart under a very low, or even negative, pressure. Arteries have thick, elastic, and muscular walls. Veins have thin, flabby walls. During periods of constipation, during straining at stool, during pregnancy, while standing upright, the slight negative pressure inside the veins is reversed. The draining function of the veins is interrupted. Blood pools within them, stagnates inside them, and pushes against their flabby walls. Wherever the vein walls are not secondarily reinforced by other tissues, bulges, bumps, and blisters develop. They look much like the blisters that develop in a defective tire.

Several things can happen next. A bulge may rupture, resulting in bleeding. A bulge may become irritated and inflamed, giving rise to itching and pain. A bulge that has repeatedly been inflamed or ruptured and then healed may become an irregularly scarred and stretched appendage. The mucous membrane covering the bulge may also become secondarily stretched and pulled out of shape and may then protrude through the anus, forming a condition known as a mucosal prolapse. The pain and discomfort from the stretched and deformed surface may cause the circular muscle of the anus to go into a spasm. The spasm of the anus is painful, too; additionally, it may cause the veins leading from the bulge to become pinched, or nipped, as if by a rubber band. Blood can then no longer circulate through the bulge and clots. The clot can become infected. The infection can erode both the vein walls and the mucous membrane covering, producing ulceration and more bleeding. And so forth, and so on.

Specific treatment, in each individual case, depends on the stage of the disease, but in general it consists of keeping the area scrupulously clean by frequent bathing in hot water, avoiding both constipation and diarrhea, using suitable ointments and creams and suppositories, and finally submitting to an operation.

One word about bleeding. While most cases of rectal bleeding are due to hemorrhoids, other diseases may be responsible. Even if you know with certainty that you suffer from hemorrhoids, there may have developed some other, unsuspected cause, as well—such as polyps, diverticulitis, proctitis, or cancer. Every case of rectal bleeding should be investigated by a doctor.

62. The Thrombosed (Clotted) Pile

This is the simplest of the misadventures that may befall the veins around the anus. The blood contained in a superficial vein clots, forms a painful, tender, hard, globular lump. Usually this lump is small—less than the size of a marble—but may be much larger.

The small thrombosed pile needs no treatment other than strict cleanliness and sitting in a hot sitz bath several times a day. The bowels must not be allowed to become constipated, and must not develop diarrhea. Read the sections in this book dealing with diet and stool softener laxatives. Avoid drastic purgatives. Avoid using any pain medication that contains constipating codeine. Avoid any other constipating medicines, such as cough and cold remedies containing codeine or its analogues. Prevent infection by washing the area with soap and water after each bowel movement (see the section on cleanliness, Section 67). Antihemorrhoidal suppositories or creams or ointments will not help in any way.

With this minimal treatment, the average-size thrombosed pile will either disappear completely or shrink into a very small, unimportant anal tag.

The very large thrombosed pile may, however, become ulcerated. It may consequently have to be cut into, so that its contained bloodclot is turned out. This is a very small operation, which your doctor can do in his office. The danger of infection is high here; attention to cleanliness (see Section 67) is most important. Hot sitz baths will help. An infection-preventing ointment (see Section 67) should be used after each sitz bath.

63. The Anal Tag

Anal tags are oval, elongated, or irregular appendages of the skin surrounding the anal orifice. They may be single, or there may be many. They are usually the end result of healed thrombosed piles (see Section 62); in effect, they are bits and tags of scar tissue. When small in size and few in number, they cause no problems whatever. When large or numerous, they are unpleasant in that they interfere with the cleansing of the anal area with toilet paper after every bowel movement. Unpleasant soiling of underwear results. They must be kept clean or they are liable to become irritated and inflamed, in which case they produce discomfort and itching. They are one of several causes of the condition known as pruritus ani (anal itch).

The single or small anal tag needs no treatment. When multiple or large, they call for washing of the area with soap and water after every bowel movement. Be careful to rinse off all traces of soap; leaving a film of soap on them is certain to produce even more irritation and itching.

Anal tags can be removed in a simple operation by your doctor either in his office or in the hospital. Your doctor may or may not need to put in stitches. Aftercare consists, once again, of strict cleanliness, hot sitz baths, and avoiding both diarrhea and constipation. Since the operation deals with the removal of scar tissue in which there are few or no nerves, there is very little pain. Healing is usually complete in a few days.

64. External and Internal Hemorrhoids—First Stage

True hemorrhoids—bulges of the rectal and anal veins—are called external if they are situated outside the anal canal and can be seen on the surface. They are called internal if they are located inside the anal canal and cannot be seen without the use of a tube-shaped instrument called a speculum. Very frequently external and internal hemorrhoids occur together.

Internal/external hemorrhoids can be present for years and give little trouble other than occasional slight discomfort and occasional slight bleeding. The bleeding usually occurs on straining at stools. The blood coats the stools but is not mixed with them. This is an important feature. Look for it. If the blood is found mostly or only as a smear on the toilet paper, then the bleeding has likely originated from external hemorrhoids. Keep in mind, however, that hemorrhoids are not the only possible cause of such bleeding.

First-stage hemorrhoids need little or no specific treatment, but cleanliness is, once again, essential to prevent irritation and infection (see Section 67). Bowel movements should be kept soft and formed; there should be neither bouts of diarrhea nor of constipation. If, as a result of an intestinal upset, you should suffer a bout of irritation, then a few sitz baths in hot water will help. You need only about three inches of hot water in your bathtub. Make it as hot as you can tolerate without scalding yourself. Sit in the tub for ten to fifteen minutes, or as long as the water will stay hot, as many times a day as you can spare the time to do so.

Antihemorrhoidal ointments and creams may help. These are described, and some are listed, in Section 67. Use a cream for application to the skin surrounding the anus, also for anal tags and for itching. Use an ointment if the problem is a prolapse of hemorrhoids from the inside of the anus.

65. External and Internal Hemorrhoids—Second Stage

Second-stage hemorrhoids regularly bulge through the anal opening on straining at stool. Consequently they bleed increasingly often and are prone to bouts of irritation and infection. By definition, hemorrhoids at this stage are reducible; that is, they can be made to retract by the effort of pelvic muscles or can be manually pushed back into the anal opening.

Second-stage hemorrhoids are decidedly more uncomfortable to live with. "Attacks of the piles" occur when a prolapsed hemorrhoidal mass is not promptly reduced; that is, when it is allowed to bulge outside the anal opening for any length of time. Such a hemorrhoidal mass is nipped by the circular muscle of the anus. It may swell and become very painful indeed. Its surface can become abraded, infected, even ulcerated.

The treatment of second-stage hemorrhoids is, once again, very strict cleanliness, attention to bowel function with prevention of both constipation and diarrhea, the use of hot sitz baths, and the use of ointments, creams, and suppositories.

In addition, every instance of a protrusion (prolapse) of a hemorrhoidal mass must be promptly reduced (pushed back) into the anal opening as soon as it occurs. "Pull back" the prolapse by prompt and strong drawing up of your pelvic muscles after every bowel movement. If you do not succeed, have a hot sitz bath, then lie down on your bed, on your left side. Lubricate your fingers with an antihemorrhoidal ointment or with vaseline. Preferably use a plastic or a rubber glove. With the flat side of your fingers, gently push and work the hemorrhoids back into the anal opening. This job cannot be rushed. A sudden push with the tips of the fingers is useless. A steady, even pressure lasting many minutes, together with a gentle rocking or massaging motion, does the trick best.

The only permanent cure of prolapsing, second-stage hemorrhoids is surgery. Sitz baths, attention to diet with avoidance of both constipation and diarrhea, the use of creams and suppositories, and the prompt pushing back of minor prolapses will allow you to plan to undergo the operation at a convenient time. Since surgery will not have to be too extensive, you will likely recover from the operation smoothly and quickly. You may get a pleasant surprise, in that the discomfort and pain following the operation may prove less than what you may have expected. Depending on the extent of the surgery, and depending also on other factors—for example, the skill of your surgeon and your own sensitivity—you may be back at your job in a week, at the very most in three to four weeks.

66. External and Internal Hemorrhoids—Third Stage

Third-stage hemorrhoids are prolapsed outside the anal opening permanently. They can at times still be pushed back, but unless continuous pressure is applied to them from the outside, they will not stay in. They are constantly abraded by underclothing. You can no longer keep yourself clean, even by the use of soap and water—in fact, the soap may now do more harm than good. Your underclothing is permanently soiled, both by fecal material and by a bloody discharge. Episodes of ulceration, of infection, become frequent. Discomfort and pain become constant. Bowel movements become experiences you dread. The relief you previously obtained from sitz baths and ointments, creams, and suppositories is now so slight as to be hardly worth the effort.

The prolapsed hemorrhoids are still subject to "attacks of the piles," but now the attacks are worse. When an extra large, previously prolapsed hemorrhoidal mass is nipped by the circular muscle of the anal canal, the spasm of the muscle may be so intense that it also nips the blood vessels leading from the area. Your hemorrhoids may swell to the size of a fist. This very unpleasant condition is known as strangulation.

An operation at this stage is urgent and may have to be performed as an emergency. It must of necessity be more extensive than if it had been performed earlier. After the operation, the recovery period may be twice as long than if the surgery had been performed electively. Even the most skillful surgeon cannot make you heal faster. You will suffer more discomfort, more pain, considerably longer.

Should you suffer from a circumferential (all the way around the anus) prolapse, then your surgeon will have to make the choice either of operating radically—of removing the whole of the prolapse all the way around and risking the complication of stenosis (circumferential scarring, which can narrow your anal opening)—or else of leaving bridges of not-too-bad hemorrhoidal tissue between excised areas. In the latter case your recovery will be quicker, but your hemorrhoids are liable to recur.

Do not unduly delay submitting to an operation. Do not wait until the third stage.

67. Living with Hemorrhoids

Eons ago, in what is today central and eastern Africa, an apelike creature with a low forehead and a potently developing brain had a sudden impulse to look around. It somehow knew, by a process of reasoning still not fully understood, that it could see better and farther if it stood up on its hind legs. It tried it once, succeeded, then tried it again. Then it decided to take a few steps in this unnatural posture.

Millions of years later this creature was given the scientific name *Homo erectus*. It achieved much—perhaps too much. But its offspring are still paying for this achievement. The bony structure of its back never adapted completely to the different stresses and strains that the erect posture brought about, so today some humans suffer from backaches. Its vascular system of arteries and veins never quite adjusted to the different fluid dynamics that the erect posture caused, and its digestive system never completely became used to the insults that food fashions made it suffer. Hence the frequency of varicose vein problems, and hence the high incidence of hemorrhoids.

It is clearly not practical for anyone to go back to walking on all fours. You cannot completely avoid the chances of developing hemorrhoids. You can, however, minimize the risks. Treat your vascular and digestive systems with kindness. Avoid gastric upsets. Avoid constipation. Avoid diarrhea. Read the sections in this book that deal with these subjects. Find out how really enjoyable it is to follow the very simple suggestions given there for eating a correctly balanced diet, planning relaxation, taking enough exercise. Do this and incidentally observe for yourself the benefits of having a truly healthy digestion. Note how much fun it is to be rid of bodily discomforts. Find out how wonderful it is to have lots of energy. Discover how your work comes easier to you, and how you can achieve more. Sense yourself smiling at people and see how they smile back. Get to know again the wonderful person with whom you once fell in love, and who is now your truly better half. Be able to cope, to manage, to get ahead in any situation.

Assume, however, that for reasons of being human you have developed symptoms of hemorrhoids. What should you do?

First, have your diagnosis confirmed by a doctor. Remember what has been repeatedly stressed in preceding sections: those symptoms may seem very typical, but they may be caused by something else. If your doctor confirms your diagnosis and does not advise you differently, follow the advice given above: make it easy for your intestine to act naturally, to produce bowel movements that are formed yet soft.

Beyond this, the cornerstone of living with hemorrhoids is strict, uncompromising cleanliness. This means, at least, daily showers, baths, or sitz baths and washing the area with soap and water after every bowel movement. Do not, however, wash with soap inside the anal canal, and make certain that you rinse off all traces of soap from the anal verge and from the surrounding area after washing.

It is simple for anyone accustomed to having regular bowel movements in the privacy of his own bathroom to get off the toilet and to step into the bathtub. It is not necessary to have a complete bath in these circumstances; just squatting in a depth of one or two inches of water is adequate. (Read further in this section about the use of ointments, and so on.)

The person who is not accustomed to having regular bowel movements at home has more of a problem. He cannot use a bathtub or shower at work. That marvelous French plumbing fixture called the bidet is almost unknown here. If you are this kind of individual, what do you do?

You can use facial tissue, but it does not work very well. More efficient are finger-protecting cleansing pads, which you can make up by simply snipping off, with scissors, triangular corner sections from ordinary, thin, polyethylene plastic bags. Each triangular corner section should be about two and a half inches in size—just large enough for you to insert the tips of your middle three fingers. Glue to one side of each such corner section, by means of a dab of a flexible latex rubber cement, an approximately four-inch by four-inch piece of surgical cotton wool, each, when not compressed, about one inch thick. (See Fig. 8) These pads are patented but are not yet in commercial production. There is no reason why you cannot make some up for your own, personal use. Keep several of them in your pocket or purse.

To use the pads, first wet two of them at the washbasin and apply soap to one. Take both pads with you into the toilet cubicle. After a bowel movement, first wipe yourself with toilet paper in the usual manner, then use the soapy pad to thoroughly wash the anal area. Drop it into the toilet bowl. Use more toilet paper to remove the excess soap. Then use the clean wet pad to wash off all traces of soap. Finally wipe or dab yourself dry with more toilet paper.

One word of caution. The pads and toilet paper together make up less bulk and contain less plastic than either feminine napkins or disposable diapers. However, if you suspect that the toilet blocks easily, flush it more than once—first before and again after you are through with the pads.

To allay the irritation and itching of anal tags, as well as to treat the perianal itching called pruritus, the best local applications are creams. For application to the prolapsed mucous membrane and for the treatment of true second- and third-stage hemorrhoids, use ointments.

The difference between creams and ointments is that creams are soluble in, and easily washed off with, water; ointments are made with a petroleum jelly base that is water resistant. You can tell the difference between them at a glance. Creams are either white or pastel; ointments are glassy gray. Creams do not interfere with skin breathing and do a better job in any situation where the skin is irritated, eczematous, or chapped. Because they are easily dissipated by sweat or body fluids, their action span is short. Ointments are greasy to the touch, will stay on the mucous membrane or skin until wiped off or deliberately washed off, and are better on normally moist mucous membrane and on prolapsed hemorrhoids.

Commercial antihemorrhoidal suppositories are commonly compounded of several ingredients, all of which are incorporated in a base of cocoa butter: coating agents so that the medication stays in one spot; balsams to hold the ingredients together; emollients (softening agents) to soften inflamed tissues; astringents to draw the tissue together (but there is no such thing as a "shrinking agent"—this is an advertising term with little real meaning); and steroids of the cortisone variety for their anti-inflammatory activity.

Some antihemorrhoidal ointments and creams also contain antibiotics, usually bacitracin, neomycin, or gentamycin. These are particularly useful in cases where the hemorrhoids are infected.

See Section 67 for suggestions about which of the three kinds of remedies to use in which stage of the hemorrhoid disease. The list of brand names that follows attempts to quote a fair selection of commercially available items. Since drug laws differ from place to place, some of the brands included here may be obtainable across the drugstore counter in some areas but dispensed only on prescription in others.

CAUTION: It is possible to develop allergies

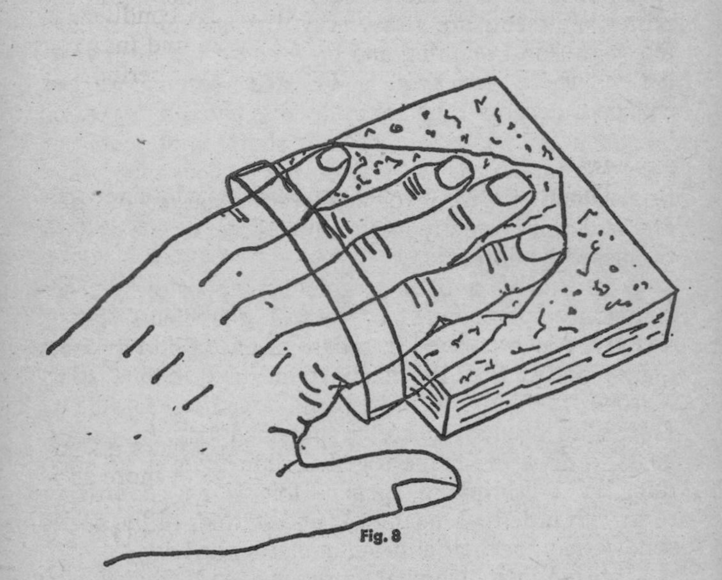

Fig. 8. Finger protecting cleansing mitt, home made from a corner of a polyethylene plastic bag. Glued to it with a dab of flexible latex cement is a pad of cotton wool.

against any of the constituents of any cream, ointment, or suppository—especially if the preparation contains antibiotics or is used too often or for too lóng a period of time. The prolonged use of antibiotics encourages the overgrowth of nonsusceptible organisms, usually but not exclusively yeasts and fungi. Too frequent use and prolonged use may result in absorbing some of the constituents into the body systems. Check with your own doctor whenever you notice that your condition is not improving or is deteriorating or if you find that you are using any preparation for prolonged periods of time.

Brands:

The following creams are said to contain cortisone or similarly acting corticosteroids: *Betnovate* (Glaxco-Allenburys) *Celestoderm V* and *Celestoderm V/2* (Schering), *Drenison* (Lilly), *Kenalog* (Squibb), *Locacorten* cream (Ciba), *Locacorten Vioform* cream (Ciba) is said also to contain Iodochlorhydroxyquin, *Medrol* (Upjohn), and *Propaderm* cream (B.D.H.).

Creams that are said to contain cortisone or a similarly acting corticosteroid as well as one or more antibiotics include: *Betnovate N* (neomycin, Glaxo-Allenburys), *Drenison cream with Neomycin* (Lilly), *Kenacomb* cream (Squibb), *Neo-Cort-Dome* cream (Dome), *Neo-Decadron* cream (M.S.D.), *Neo-Medrol* cream (Upjohn), and *Valisone G* cream (gentamycin) (Schering).

Ointments that are said to contain cortisone or similarly acting corticosteroids include: *Betnovate* (Glaxo-Allenburys), *Drenison* (Lilly), *Kenalog* (Squibb), *Locacorten* (Ciba), *Locacorten Vioform* (with iodochlorhydroxyquin); (Ciba), *Propaderm* (B.D.H.).

Ointments said to contain both cortisone or a similarly acting corticosteroid, and one or more antibiotics include: *Betnovate N* (neomycin; Glaxo-Allenburys), *Drenison Ointment with Neomycin* (Lilly), *Kenacomb* (Squibb), *Neo-Cortef* (Upjohn), and *Valisone G* (Schering).

The following ointments and suppositories are said to be specifically formulated for the treatment of hemorrhoids. Most are complex formulations containing soothing agents, balsams, coating agents, astringents, and so on: *Alcos-Anal* ointment and suppositories (Denver), *Anusol* ointment and suppositories (Warner Chilcott), *Hemoral* ointment and suppositories (M. & M.), and *Wyanoids* ointment and suppositories (Wyeth).

The following preparations are said to contain additional local anesthetics: *Hemroydine* ointment and suppositories (Dow), *P.N.S.* suppositories (Winthrop), *Nupercainal* cream, ointment, and suppositories (Ciba) and *Xylocaine* ointment, suppositories, and spray (Astra).

The following are said to contain cortisone or a similarly acting corticosteroid: *Anugesic HC* ointment and suppositories (Warner Chilcott) and *Wyanoids HC* suppositories (Wyeth).

One preparation is said to contain a corticosteroid, a local anesthetic, and an antibiotic: *Proctosedyl* ointment and suppositories (Roussel).

Part VI. Flatulence

68. Introduction

As was described in Section 2, the normal intestinal tract, from the time of birth on, always contains some intestinal gas. Most of this gas is derived from swallowed air. Every time you swallow anything—food, drink, saliva—you swallow some air with it. Some people swallow much more air than others.

The gas you have in your stomach is just about pure air. Farther along in the small intestine, where food is being churned into a nutrient mash, the swallowed air contains volatile products of fermentation. Still farther along in the colon, the air-gas mixture also contains volatile products of putrefaction.

The chemical composition of normal small intestinal gas is as follows:

Nitrogen	c.70%
Oxygen	10–12%
Carbon dioxide	6–9%
Hydrogen	1–3%
Hydrogen sulfide	1–10%
Volatile basic groups (ammonia, methane, amines, etc.)	0.5–5%

Large intestinal (colonic) gas contains less carbon dioxide but more hydrogen sulfide. It is the latter—which you may remember from your chemistry class at school as having the smell of rotten eggs—that makes flatus offensive.

Fortunate indeed is the person who never suffers from the discomfort of gas distension or from the misery of bloating. He is not only fortunate but also unique. Excessive distension and bloating are very common afflictions.

The most frequent cause of recurring, nagging, almost constant "gas" problems is excessive swallowing of air. Just like rubbing one's nose or constantly tugging at one's ear, gulping air can be a habit. Like any habit, once air swallowing is fully ingrained it can be difficult to eradicate. What is more, most people who suffer from this habit are completely unaware of it. Do relatives, friends, and neighbors notice? Rarely.

The second common cause of excessive air swallowing originates in some minor, transient intestinal upset or spasm that makes you gulp air and try to burp. The normal, physiological mechanism of voluntary burping is such that to accomplish a voluntary burp you must first swallow a mouthful of air "halfway down." This then stimulates your diaphragm and abdominal muscles into a short, sharp contraction. Swallowing a mouthul of air in this manner amounts to "pump priming." Your subconscious hopes that the resultant burp will expel both the air you have gulped down to prime the pump and a portion of the air distending your stomach already. Too often, however, instead of expelling stomach air, each forced burp adds more. Instead of getting relief, your distension increases.

Note, however, that an involuntary, nonforced burp does not involve the swallowing of air first and does relieve distension.

Voluntary forced burping can also become a habit and commonly coexists with the air swallowing habit. A person so afflicted usually feels quite well in the morning, after a good night's sleep. As the day wears on, the constant air gulping and forced burping combine and produce more and more distension, more and more discomfort. The problem becomes acute after meals. If a sufferer is subjected to mental or emotional stress, the result is misery.

If you suffer from "gas trouble" that is due to habitual air swallowing and forced burping, the first thing to do, obviously, is to stop. Chances are, however, that you are not aware of what you are doing. The thing to do then is to ask someone who shares your life with you to watch you. Tell that person that you will appreciate it if he will draw your attention to it every time he notices you taking a gulp of air. Tell this person further, and mean it, that you will not be offended and that you will definitely not think of it as nagging. Learn to recognize your problem. Learn first to catch yourself in the act, then learn to avoid the act.

The next thing to do in these circumstances is to take extra exercise. Exercise relaxes the circular gate muscles (sphincter muscles) that separate various segments of the intestinal tract. Exercise stimulates the intestinal movements called peristalsis. It helps to prevent gas from building up pressure in any one area. After abdominal operations, patients who insist on lying still in bed suffer from distension, flatulence, and constipation. Once they get out of bed and march up and down the hospital corridor, their gas troubles vanish. So get out of your armchair. Switch off your TV. Choose any type or kind of exercise that appeals to you, but do it regularly. At the very least, take brisk walks daily. If you cannot decide on what to do, if you have almost grown roots, get some help from music. Do calisthenics to music or, better still, put on a modern rock record. Do not worry if you have never danced to rock before. Just stand on your living room rug with your feet slightly apart and pretend that you are drying your back with a beach towel. Vigorously. Do it in tune to the rock . . . and revel in the relief you get.

Finally, if you are still looking for relief, read the section on flatulence and spice, at the end of this part.

69. Flatulence as a Symptom of Illness

Apart from habitual air swallowing and voluntary forced burping, flatulence is not an ailment by itself. Like diarrhea and constipation, it is a symptom. Symptoms are what you yourself feel or experience. Signs of disease are what an observer, usually a doctor, can see, hear, or feel on your body.

There are a multiplicity of illnesses, some serious and some not so serious, of which flatulence is one of the symptoms. Other symptoms not only coexist in these illnesses but often overshadow it. Only some of the many illnesses are listed here. None of them is suitable for self-treatment. Consult your doctor and follow his advice if you think that you suffer from any of them.

Gastrointestinal Tract

A condition of spasm that afflicts the large bowel has already been extensively dealt with in the sections of this book that deal with spastic colitis (Section 48) prediverticulosis, and diverticular disease (Section 49). Flatulence is a part of the disease picture of all of these.

The upper gastrointestinal tract is subject to spasm, too. Spasms of the esophagus occur in some people. The gas-bloat syndrome is a disease entity in which the junction of the esophagus with the stomach is so tight that ordinary (involuntary) burping is almost impossible. Spasms of the stomach proper are part of several acute illnesses, such as food poisoning, gastritis, and gastroenteritis, and can occur as the result of overeating or follow acute intoxication with drugs or alcohol. More prolonged and chronic spasms of the whole or parts of the stomach and duodenum are a feature of some stages of the formation of peptic ulcers. Small intestinal spasm likewise occurs, uncommonly, as a feature of an illness that afflicts the small intestine principally, more often as the result of adhesions and following inflammations of other organs that in turn involve the small bowel.

Liver, Gall Bladder, and Pancreas

Excessive flatulence is a symptom of gallstones and a doctor investigating your gas problem will probably order x-rays of the gall bladder. Spasms of the pancreas (sweatbread) have been alluded to already in Section 24, on booze.

The Heart and Lungs

Certain kinds of heart disease cause the biliary tract (the liver, bile channels, and gall bladder) to react with spasms, which then secondarily afflict the intestinal tract, thus producing flatulence. Cardiac angina (a type of heart pain that occurs on muscular exertion) is one. A heart attack (coronary artery thrombosis) is another.

Sufferers from asthma commonly experience flatulence during attacks of this disease, as the result of swallowing air while laboring to breathe.

70. Flatulence and Diet

Eating an unbalanced diet is apt to result in many problems, some of which have been described already in the sections dealing with diarrhea and with constipation. Excessive fermentation results from a diet that contains too much carbohydrate. The resultant gas is acid. The treatment of this condition is to eat less sugar and fewer bakery goods, sweets, potatoes, corn, and macaroni. Excessive putrefaction is produced by a diet too high in protein. This sort of diet is expensive and, after a while, hardly palatable. Excessive putrefaction does occur in some people after they have indulged in a heavy dinner. More frequently, such problems afflict people who depend for most of their protein requirements on vegetables—peas, lentils, beans, nuts, soybeans. The inhabitants of India, Mexico, and other hot countries discovered ages ago that most of the ill effects of such vegetarian diets can be prevented and rectified by the plentiful use of spices.

71. Flatulence and Spice

Whatever the cause of flatulence, in addition to the remedies mentioned in Section 70 there exist means of prevention and treatment so ancient that they are part of the human cultural heritage. These mouthwatering items are known by many names. Doctors call them carminatives, or stomachics. Pharmacologists call their active principles essential aromatic volatile oils. Cooks and housewives call them condiments and spices.

The following list is by no means complete. You should have no trouble adding to it:

Anise	Liquorice
Bay	Menthol
Bitters (various kinds)	Mustard
Caraway	Myrrh
Cinnamon	Nutmeg
Chili (a mixture)	Onion
Cloves	Orange peel
Curry (a mixture)	Pepper (many kinds)
Dill	Peppermint (and other mints)
Eucalyptus	Rosemary
Ginger	Thyme
Lemon peel	Valerian

The essential volatile aromatic oils contained in spices are, when pure, strong antiseptics and potent tissue irritants. In low concentrations they are aromatic food-flavoring agents. They tempt the sense of smell.

They increase salivation. They augment the appetite. They serve to increase the flow of digestive juices. They check the growth of yeasts and of other gas-producing, fermentation, and putrefaction agents. They lessen the intensity of stomach and intestinal peristaltic cramps and relax the tightness of intestinal sphincters, thus easing burping. Like caffeine, the active ingredient of coffee, they even have a stimulant effect on the brain.

It is not surprising that food served as part of special festive fare is almost always well seasoned. Condiments and spices make the meal. They alone enable the average person, with the average stomach, to eat his way through several courses of a meal that would otherwise be far too filling. What is surprising is that sufferers from flatulence have not discovered, long ago, that seasoning will also improve the digestion of ordinary, everyday meals.

There is a difference between highly spiced foods and properly seasoned foods. Hot Indian curry and Tabasco sauce are not for everybody. Rare, however, is the person who cannot stomach foods gently seasoned with a little cinnamon or rosemary or who cannot eat a mint candy or enjoy a delicately scented after-dinner liqueur.

If you suffer from indigestion with flatulence, and if you doctor does not advise you differently, get away from canned or frozen TV dinners. Go easy on the type of fast, precooked, ready-to-eat foods that taste like cotton wool, with the cotton removed. Live a little. Enjoy your cooking, and revel in the sensation of how your intestinal tract enjoys it too.

72. Suggestions for Simple-to-Make Seasoned Foods

Breakfasts

Orange juice. Tomato juice with a dash of Worcester sauce. Cinnamon toast or waffle. Cinnamon baked apple. Chilled prunes sprinkled with cinnamon. Pineapple spiked with cloves. Smoked salmon on caraway rye bread. Orange slices with mint jelly. Spiced omelettes (many kinds).

Lunches

Spinach soufflé with rosemary. Spiced cheeses on caraway rye bread. Mint sherbets. Cucumber yoghurt with mint. Ginger-flavored shrimp on toast. Orange cake. Mint pears. Banana bread with lemon peel. Anise cakes. Gingerbread.

Dinners

Stews flavored with thyme. Apple pie with nutmeg. Ham studded with cloves. Chili con carne. Italian meatballs (many spices). Spumoni. Meat loaf with rosemary. Roast lamb with mint. Lemon meringue pie.

Sweets and Candies

Peppermint, spearmint, other mints. Liquorice. Ginger.

Liqueurs

Creme de Menthe, Kummel, Cointreau, Pernod, Benedictine, many others.

Index